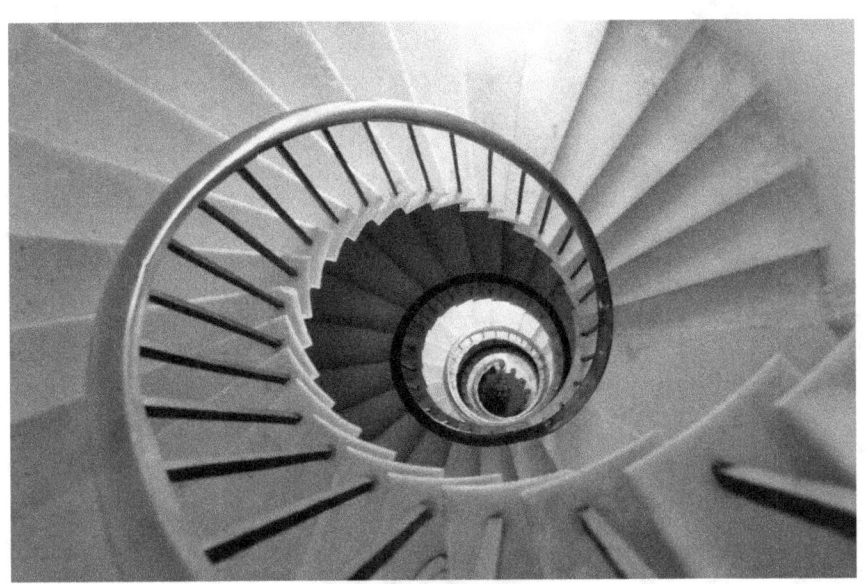

Vertigo RX:
Understanding and Managing Vertigo - A Practical Guide

Timothy D. Frantz, MD
Matthew Kim, MD

Copyright © 2024

All rights reserved. In accordance with the U.S. copyright Act of 1976, the scanning, uploading, and electronic sharing of any part of this book without the permission of the publisher constitute unlawful piracy and theft of the author's intellectual property. If you would like to use material from the book (other than for review purposes), prior written permission must be obtained by contacting the publisher at VertigoRxBook@gmail.com

Thank you for your support of the author's rights.

Kindle Direct Publishing

First Edition: June 2024

Library of Congress Cataloging-in-Publication Data

Frantz, Timothy

Kim, Matthew

Vertigo / Timothy Frantz, etal. – 1st ed.

192 pp. 15.24x22.86 cm.

Includes bibliographical references and index.

Library of Congress control number: in application

ISBN 9798327399198

1. Dizziness. 2. Vertigo. 3. Dizziness Treatment. 4. Vertigo treatment.

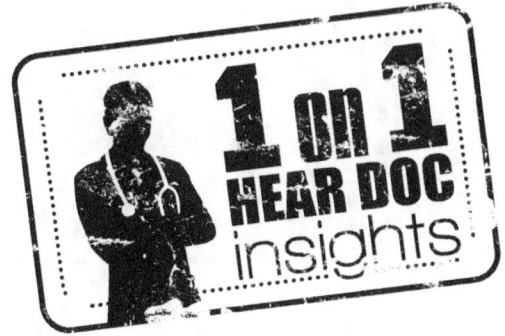

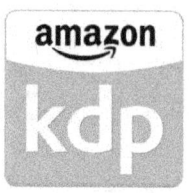
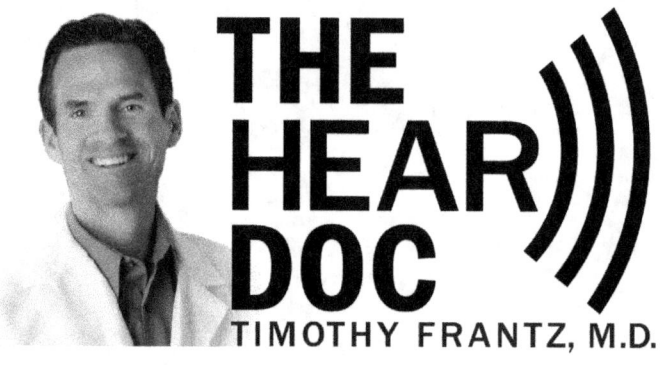

Vertigo RX: Understanding and Managing Vertigo - A Practical Guide

Timothy D. Frantz, MD
Matthew Kim, MD

DISCLAIMER

This publication is intended to provide educational, helpful, informative material. It is not intended to diagnose, treat, cure, or prevent any health problems, vertigo, dizziness, hearing loss condition, nor is intended to replace the advice of a licensed medical professional. No action should be taken solely on the contents of this book. Always consult a qualified health-care professional on any matters regarding vertigo or hearing loss, and before adopting any suggestions or drawing inferences from the content of this book.

The authors and publisher specifically disclaim all responsibility for any liability, loss or risk, personal or otherwise, which is incurred as a consequence, directly or indirectly, from the use, adoption or application of any contents of this book without the recommendation of a qualified professional.

Any and all product names referenced within this book are the trademarks of their respective owners. None of these owners have sponsored, authorized, endorsed, or approved this book. Always read all information provided by the manufacturer before using any medication/device/product. The authors and publishers are not responsible for claims made by manufacturers. The statements made in this book have not been evaluated by the United States Food and Drug Administration, and are solely based on the authors' cumulative research, and over 35 years combined experience of Dr. Timothy Frantz and Dr. Matthew Kim's experience working as an otolaryngologist and as an Otolaryngology resident.

DEDICATION

We dedicate this book to over 40 million people in the United States who suffer from vertigo and/or hearing loss. Vertigo, dizziness and balance-related conditions are among the most common health problems in U.S. adults. Nearly 40 percent of adults in the U.S. experience vertigo at least once in their lifetime.

This book is also dedicated to Rosalind Franklin University of Medicine and Science, **The Chicago Medical School**, in North Chicago, Illinois. As an alumnus and a current medical student, we are grateful to be a part of this school that provided an exceptional education and most importantly believed in us to pursue our passion to help those with ear disease such as vertigo and hearing loss.

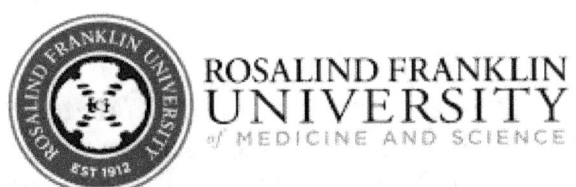

ACKNOWLEDGEMENTS

We would like to express our gratitude to the many people who sustained us while we wrote this book; to all those who provided support, offered comments, and assisted in the editing, proofreading and design. We would also like to thank Dean Archana Chatterjee, MD, PhD and her staff of professionals at RFU/The Chicago Medical School for their encouragement and facilitation of this book.

Above all we want to thank our families. They supported and encouraged us in spite of all the time it took us away from them.

Contents

Preface   p 15

Callouts   p 17

STEP 1-

The Basics (What is Vertigo?)

Chapter 1: The Importance of Good Balance   p 23

Chapter 2: Achieving Normal Balance   p 30

Chapter 3: Dizziness versus True Vertigo:
Deciphering the Discrepancies   p 39

Chapter 4: Common Causes of Vertigo   p 44

Chapter 5: Recognizing Critical Signs:
When to Seek Urgent Medical Attention   p 56

STEP 2-

The Diagnosis (Complete Medical History, Examination and Testing)

Chapter 6: The Comprehensive Medical History in Vertigo Assessment p 62

Chapter 7: Physical Examination for Patients with Vertigo p 70

Chapter 8: Understanding Vertigo Tests p 81

Chapter 9: Ophthalmological (Eye-related) Causes of Vertigo p 110

STEP 3 -

The Treatments (Dietary, Medicinal, Physical Therapeutics, Surgical, and Others)

Chapter 10: Navigating Treatment Options for Dizziness and Vertigo p 115

Chapter 11: Physical Therapy for Vertigo p 120

Chapter 12: Dietary Treatments for Vertigo p 124

Chapter 13: Medicinal Treatments for Vertigo: An Overview p 131

Chapter 14: Physical Therapy for Vertigo:
Regain Your Balance and Confidence   p 135

Chapter 15: Surgical Treatments for Vertigo:
Exploring Your Options   p 139

Chapter 16: Assistive Devices for Vertigo   p 147

Chapter 17: Driving Considerations with Vertigo   p 152

STEP 4 -

The Beginning (Not the End)

Chapter 18: Understanding Vertigo:
A Summary of Treatment Goals   p 159

Chapter 19: The Future of Vertigo Treatments,
Diagnosis and Prevention of Falls and Injury   p 166

Chapter 20: Final Thoughts   p 175

Glossary of Terms   p 177

References   p 181

The Hear Doc's ™ other books   p 189

ABOUT THE AUTHORS p 191

Preface

If you need help with dizziness or vertigo, you have already taken the first step by buying this book. Our goal is to give you helpful and clear advice and the tools you need to help identify if you have vertigo. Hopefully, we can also help you decide if professional medical help is required, understand the causes, diagnosis, and treatment of vertigo and balance disorders.

You will:
- **Learn about dizziness and vertigo**
- **Recognize if you have vertigo**
- **Understand the importance of professional medical evaluation**
- **Learn safety tips for patients with vertigo**
- **Learn how to navigate often confusing advice**
- **Learn about serious causes of vertigo**

- **Discover the <u>4 Steps to Relief</u>**

Unfortunately, vertigo is a common problem. We wrote this book to educate and inform the reader about vertigo, its common causes, diagnostic testing, and potential treatments. It is our hope that this book will help you determine the next steps, and most importantly, know when to seek medical care. Our purpose is NOT to write a comprehensive medical text, but an easy-to-read, clear, simple explanation of what may be going on when vertigo occurs, and what can be done about it.

According to the Cleveland Clinic up to 40% of Americans experience one or more episodes of vertigo during their lifetime. Although it can occur at any age, it is much more common in those 65 years or older, and is also more common in women.
According to the Merriam-Webster's Dictionary, vertigo is defined as "a sensation of motion in which the individual's surroundings seem to whirl dizzily."

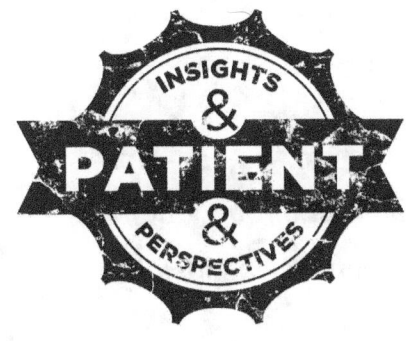
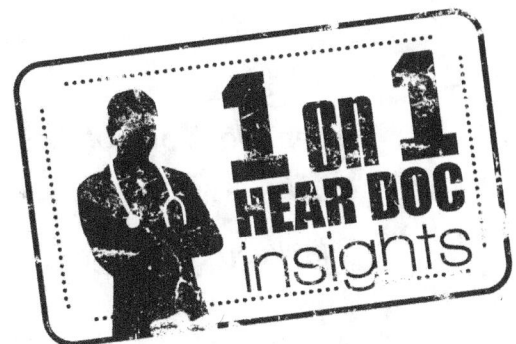
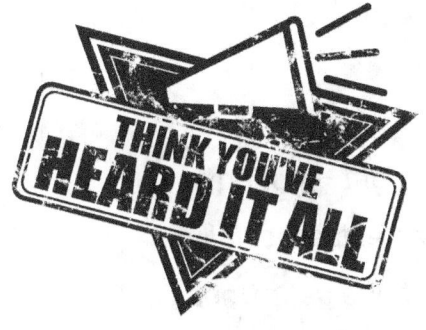
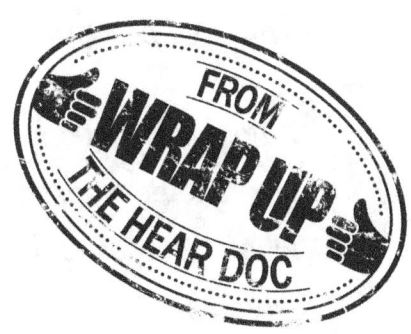

Keep a look out for these **callouts** *throughout the book to get unique perspectives and insights that keep you turning pages….*

Welcome to a Conversation with The Hear Doc ™!

Alright, let's get one thing straight – nobody wants to be stuck in a snoozefest, especially when it comes to health stuff. We get it; medical jargon can be as thrilling as watching paint dry. But fear not, because this book is not your typical medical monologue. We're here to chat, not lecture.

Throughout our little journey together, keep an eye out for our special callouts. They're like the rockstars of information, and they go by some fancy names:

- *Think You've Heard it All:*
    - *Brace yourself for tales that might make you go, "Wait, what?" Life is full of surprises, and so is this book.*
- *One-On-One Hear Doc Insights:*
    - *Ever wished you could pick a doctor's brain without the hassle? Well, here's your chance. Get cozy with some one-on-one insights straight from The Hear Doc ™*
- *Patient Insights & Perspectives:*
    - *Let's throw in some real stories, shall we? Because sometimes, the best lessons come from those who've been there, done that.*
- *Wrap Up from The Hear Doc ™!*
    - *Time to tie it all together. Consider this your grand finale, a wrap-up that'll leave you thinking, "I'm so glad I picked up this book."*

So, why the chatty vibe? We want to make sure this isn't just another textbook you'll forget about. Our mission? To make you the vertigo expert at your next trivia night. Just kidding! But seriously, we want you to finish this book feeling like you've had a good conversation about vertigo. No fancy diplomas or white coats – just a friendly conversation.

Our goal? To answer your burning questions, squash those vertigo myths, and nudge you in the right direction. After all, we're not just here to talk; we want you to take the next step. Go ahead, schedule that appointment with a local healthcare professional who can guide you through this dizzying journey.

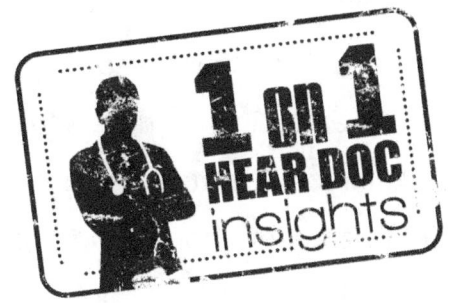

The symptoms of vertigo can be incredibly distressing. Patients frequently experience a sudden sensation of spinning, falling, or losing balance, often accompanied by profuse sweating, intense nausea, vomiting, and blurred or double vision. These alarming symptoms can make it feel like a stroke or heart attack, prompting many to urgently seek medical attention. This book is dedicated to addressing these urgent concerns and providing clarity and relief.

Why should you read our book?

We understand the frustration of wading through medical jargon in countless books and articles, only to end up more confused. Our book is different. As a medical student and a board-certified Otolaryngologist, we empathize with you and aim to present information in a clear, straightforward manner. This book is designed for everyday readers curious about vertigo and those seeking help. You may have normal balance and no dizziness and picked up this book looking for answers to help you cope with a family member or friend with vertigo. While we're still learning ourselves, we've had the invaluable guidance of Dr. Timothy Frantz, who brings over 30 years of experience to this project. By the conclusion of this book, you'll not only understand vertigo better but also feel more equipped to manage it effectively, and seek appropriate care.

Chapter 1

The Importance of Good Balance

What is Balance?

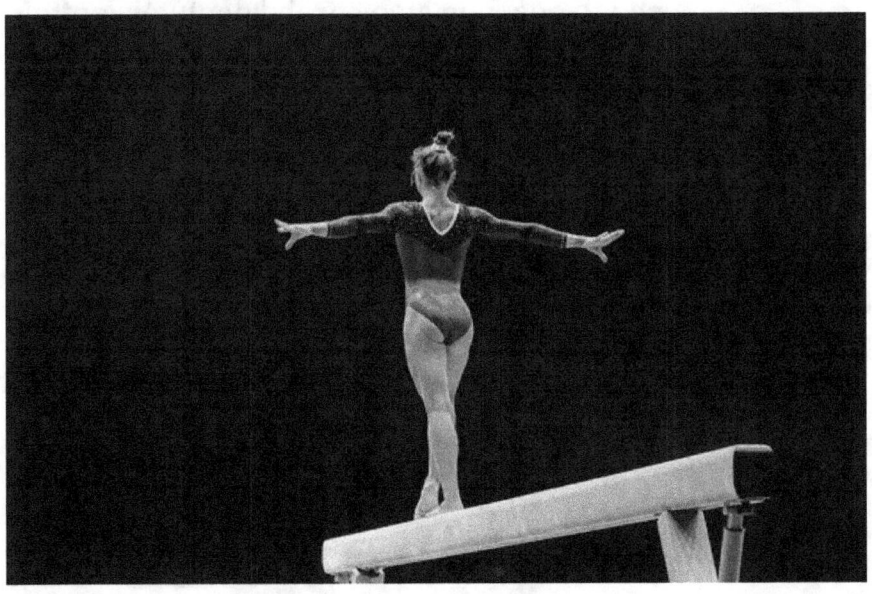

When we think of the word balance, what comes to mind? I'm sure some may think of a balance beam, a balance scale, or even some standing on one foot and not falling over. Well it can be a noun or a verb. In terms of using balance as a verb, medical school always emphasized, "You need to have a work-life balance." We agree that is necessary, however, in the field of clinical health, it more relates to someone standing on one foot. In essence it is used to describe stability and postural control (Pollock et al., 2000).

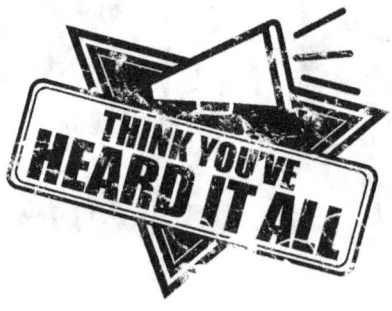

Fun fact: Despite many using the term, "balance," there is no universally accepted definition of human balance (Pollock et al., 2000).

Why is it important?

Understanding balance is crucial as it profoundly impacts our daily lives. In the context of health, doctors utilize this concept extensively when evaluating patients. It prompts the question: how exactly does balance assist doctors in a patient evaluation? Balance serves as a key indicator of brain function, potential bone and spine issues, and even ear disorders in patients.

Without good balance, we would struggle to perform activities independently, constantly facing the risk of falling during our daily routines. Regrettably, this is particularly prevalent among older adults. The increased risks of falling impairs quality of life and creates physical limitations in many older adults (Dunsky, 2019).

- Sprains and strains are often caused by a lack of balance. Balance is essential for every movement we make, and poor balance increases the risk of injuries such as ankle sprains.

- A healthy balance system provides more energy and strength, which enhances your ability to move freely and confidently. This is especially crucial for individuals with health issues such as dizziness. Maintaining good balance not only helps prevent falls but also improves overall mobility and quality of life. Research indicates that balance exercises, such as tai chi or yoga, can be particularly effective in enhancing stability and reducing symptoms of vertigo and dizziness. For instance, a study published in the journal "NeuroRehabilitation" in 2016 demonstrated that participants who engaged in regular balance training showed significant improvements in their ability to maintain equilibrium and experienced fewer episodes of dizziness. Therefore, prioritizing balance exercises is essential for anyone looking to improve their physical health and well-being.

What happens when we lose balance or the ability to balance?

Do you remember the time you spun around in a circle multiple times and then lost your balance and fell to the ground? That sensation you felt is known as dizziness. Dizziness can encompass a range of sensations, including light-headedness, faintness, feeling woozy, and being off-balance.

When we lose our balance, falling is a common outcome. However, when people completely lose their ability to stay stable, they may experience the sensation of the world spinning, floating, or a falling sensation of movement, which is known as vertigo. This can lead to more severe consequences. In such cases, people might experience dizziness **and** vertigo, where it feels like the world is spinning around them.

How can balance help with dizziness and vertigo?

Research suggests that improving your balance through specific exercises can help with vertigo. Studies have shown that balance exercises, like standing on one leg with your eyes closed can significantly improve stability (Chang et al., 2008). This improvement in balance may also help reduce dizziness and vertigo.

Chapter 2

Achieving Normal Balance

Balance indicates the capacity to sustain the body's center of gravity over its base of support (Shumway-Cook & Woollacott, 2001). This equilibrium is established through a sophisticated sensorimotor control system incorporating inputs from vision, proprioception (how your feet and spine feel the floor), and the vestibular system, the latter being a specialized system that manages spatial orientation and motion, harmonizing its signals towards the brain. The brain, in turn, integrates this diverse information and communicates it to the eyes and muscles of the body (Vestibular Disorder Association et al., 2016). Basically, many parts of our body help contribute towards sustaining balance.

One critical contributor to our balance is our vision. Closing your eyes and attempting to walk may result in instability, emphasizing that eyes serve not only to perceive what lies ahead but also to gauge the spatial arrangement of everything around. This visual input allows the eyes to transmit vital information to the brain, aiding in orienting ourselves relative to other objects, particularly our own position.

Another example that contributes to the body's balance is our muscles and joints are equipped with sensory receptors attuned to stretch or pressure, heightening awareness of our surroundings. Consider the scenario of closing your eyes – with the loss of visual spatial awareness, your lower body must adapt to the environment to prevent falls and maintain spatial awareness. Changes are detected by muscles and joints, which relay this information to the brain.

Many know that the function of the ear is to allow one to hear sound. But astonishingly the ear does more than just that. It is one of the major components for our sense of balance. There are three parts that make up the ear. The outer, middle, and inner ear. The inner ear has a special balance organ that makes up the vestibular system which is the system that helps us achieve balance. It consists of 3 semicircular canals and 2 otolith organs, known as the utricle and saccule. These canals and organs contain specialized fluid.

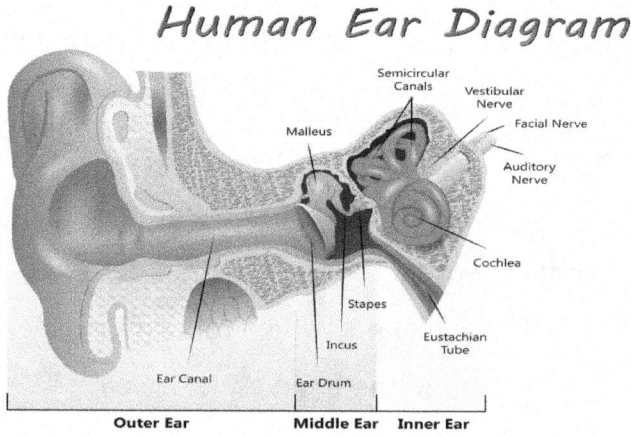

Each of the **semicircular canals** contain a tiny valve called a "cupula." The cupula is a gelatinous membrane with specialized sensory cells in it. Now remember there is fluid inside these canals as well. So whenever we move our heads, the fluid inside these canals will also move. As the fluid moves, the cupulas inside the canals sway along too. You can imagine coral at the bottom of the ocean swaying in whatever direction the current takes it. When these valves sway, they will activate and send signals to the brain by means of nerves. There are 3 canals (superior, horizontal, and posterior) and each one responds to rotational acceleration according to the direction your head moves. Therefore, one canal may respond when your head moves up and down, another when your head rotates left to right, and the third when tilting your head left and right.

The **otolith organs** (utricle and saccule) are found diagonally under the semicircular canals and have similar functions as the canals. The organs contain sensory cells as well. The difference between the two is that the cells are encased in a membrane embedded with tiny crystals called otoliths or "ear rocks." These otoliths have mass (weight) and are responsible for detecting gravitational acceleration, such as when you are in an elevator. As you go up or down in an elevator, the small rocks will activate and send signals towards the brain. In the brain the information is coordinated and signals are relayed to the eyes, joints, or muscles. This is how our bodies allow us to keep our balance and grasp our bearings.

Normal physical balance is achieved through a combination of sensory input, muscular coordination, and the body's ability to adjust and maintain equilibrium. Here are some key factors that contribute to achieving and maintaining physical balance:

Sensory Input:

Being mindful of movements and focusing on balance can help prevent falls or accidents. Paying attention to changes in your body's position and making subtle adjustments can prevent imbalance. Since balance is achieved through a complex system that receives information from our eyes, brain, muscles, joints, and vestibular organs, it's imperative to be aware that a slight dysfunction in any of these inputs can cause imbalance.

Healthy Lifestyle:

General health factors such as maintaining a healthy weight, staying hydrated, and getting adequate sleep can contribute to your body's overall functionality. As people age, balance might naturally decline due to changes in sensory system, muscle mass, or even bone density. However, a study showed that being physically active can promote balance for young and older adults which can ultimately help prevent age-related decline of postural balance performance (Sarto et al., 2022).

They say an apple a day keeps the doctor away, it's not entirely wrong. It just needs to include adequate physical activity and sleep!

Footwear:

According to Gabell et al., heel elevation has been associated with a greater risk of falling in older people. Therefore, wearing lower heel shoes or flats can help prevent that from happening. It was also found in another study that there was an inverse correlation of shoe heel height to balance and efficiency of walking. In other words, the higher the heel height the worse your balance and walking will be (Weon & Cha, 2018). Many patients feel that they should walk barefoot to reduce fall risk, however, particularly in older folks, the opposite is true. They have grown up wearing shoes daily for many decades and fall risk is significantly greater walking barefoot.

According to Julie Shein and the Vestibular Disorders Association the recommended heel height for shoes is 2.7 cm or less. Another factor to keep in mind is the hardness of the sole. Older people's balance and proprioception (the ability to feel the ground under your feet) is worse in shoes with a thick, soft midsole (Robbins et al). Shoes with a soft sole caused more imbalance since they require an increase in muscle activation to maintain their balance (Perry et al).

With that said, older adults should wear a shoe with a thin, hard sole to improve your balance.

Balance is a complex interplay of various factors, and maintaining balance is an ongoing process. If you're concerned about your balance, it's a good idea to consult with a healthcare professional or a physical therapist for personalized advice and exercises.

Chapter 3

Dizziness versus True Vertigo: Deciphering the Discrepancies

Dizziness and vertigo are terms often used interchangeably to describe sensations of imbalance or unsteadiness. However, these experiences stem from distinct origins and manifest in different ways. This chapter delves into the nuances that differentiate dizziness from true vertigo, exploring their definitions, causes, and accompanying symptoms.

Defining Dizziness:

Dizziness is a broad term encompassing various sensations, including lightheadedness, unsteadiness, and a general feeling of being off-balance. Individuals experiencing dizziness may describe a sensation of floating, wooziness, or a feeling that their surroundings are spinning. Dizziness can be caused by a multitude of factors, ranging from dehydration, low blood sugar, stress, and even certain medications.

Types of Dizziness:

> Presyncope: This type of dizziness is often described as feeling faint or on the verge of passing out. It is commonly associated with conditions like low blood pressure, hypoxia, dehydration, or orthostatic hypotension.
> Disequilibrium: Individuals with disequilibrium experience a general sense of unsteadiness or imbalance, as though they might fall. This type of dizziness is frequently linked to musculoskeletal or neurological issues.

Defining True Vertigo:

True vertigo, on the other hand, is a more specific and intense experience characterized by a false sense of rotational movement, either of oneself or the environment. The perception of spinning or whirling can be severe and is often accompanied by nausea and vomiting. True vertigo typically originates from disturbances in the vestibular system, which includes the inner ear and its connections to the brain.

Causes of True Vertigo:

>Inner Ear Disorders (Peripheral Vertigo): Conditions such as benign paroxysmal positional vertigo (BPPV), vestibular neuritis, and Meniere's disease can induce true vertigo by affecting the normal functioning of the inner ear.

Central Nervous System Disorders (Central Vertigo): Certain neurological conditions, such as migraines, multiple sclerosis, tumors impacting the brainstem, and even strokes can also lead to true vertigo.

Distinguishing Features:

One key method to differentiate between dizziness and true vertigo is to inquire about the nature of the sensation. While dizziness may involve a feeling of light-headedness or unsteadiness, true vertigo is characterized by a vivid perception of spinning, floating, falling, or rotational movement. In other words, if you are not moving but the whole room is spinning then most likely you are experiencing true vertigo.

In summary, understanding the disparities between dizziness and true vertigo is crucial for accurate diagnosis and effective management. Whether caused by peripheral vestibular disorders, central nervous system abnormalities, or other factors, recognizing the distinct characteristics of each condition is a crucial step toward providing appropriate medical intervention and improving the overall well-being of individuals experiencing these symptoms.

Chapter 4

Common Causes of Vertigo

Vertigo, a disconcerting sensation of dizziness characterized by a false perception of movement, can arise from a myriad of underlying causes. It is imperative to recognize the multifaceted nature of vertigo, and seeking professional medical advice is paramount for accurate diagnosis and effective management. This chapter provides an in-depth examination of various common causes of vertigo, shedding light on their distinct characteristics and manifestations.

Benign Paroxysmal Positional Vertigo (BPPV):

- Description: BPPV stands as one of the foremost contributors to peripheral vestibular vertigo with

a prevalence of ~2%. Females are 2-3x more likely to be affected by this condition than males (Kim & Zee, 2014).
- Clinical Features: It occurs very suddenly and typically only lasts less than a minute. A common trigger is from rotating your head or changing head positions quickly.
- Mechanism: Caused by the displacement of minute calcium crystals within the inner ear, BPPV disrupts the normal balance signals.
- Analogy: Imagine carrying a substantial bucket of water. Tilting the bucket leads to a shift in water balance, akin to the inner ear disturbance in BPPV. Attempts to correct this

imbalance exacerbate instability, creating a cycle of vertigo.

Vestibular Neuritis:

- Description: Vestibular neuritis involves inflammation of the vestibular nerve, impacting spatial orientation and balance. This is usually caused by a previous viral upper respiratory infection. It is the second most common cause of peripheral vertigo after BPPV (Muncie et al., 2017). Affecting males and females equally (Kim, 2020).
- Clinical Features: Sudden onset of severe vertigo, often accompanied by nausea and imbalance. This condition is distinguished by a constant

sensation of vertigo that can last for a couple days to sometimes even several weeks or months.
- Analogy: Imagine you jammed your toe. Later that toe starts to swell up, turn red and hot. This similar mechanism is happening in your vestibular nerve causing dysfunction.

Meniere's Disease:

- Description: A chronic disorder of the inner ear characterized by recurring vertigo, hearing loss, and tinnitus. It is more common in females than males (Basura et al., 2020).
- Mechanism: Imbalance in inner ear fluid regulation (too much

inner ear fluid) is believed to contribute to the symptoms.
- Clinical Features: It can cause a triad of peripheral vertigo, tinnitus (ringing of the ears), and asymmetric sensorineural hearing loss, or feeling of "plugged" ears. These episodes can last for several hours. Many patients express ear fullness with this condition.
- Analogy: Imagine boiling a tea kettle. When you boil a tea kettle it creates a lot of pressure causing it to make a loud sound. All that pressure is occuring in the inner ear as well, which may help to explain these symptoms.

Migraine-Associated Vertigo (MAV)Vestibular Migraine:

- Description: Peripheral vertigo as a symptom of migraines, extending beyond the typical headache presentation. In order to be diagnosed with vestibular migraines you need to at least present with 5 episodes of vestibular symptoms lasting 5 minutes to 72 hours (Hilton et al.,2024).
- Mechanism: Currently the mechanism of how vestibular migraines occur is up for debate but may be associated with blood vessel spasms.
- Manifestations: Episodes of vertigo may be accompanied by

visual disturbances and sensitivity to light.

Acoustic Neuroma:

- Description: A benign tumor derived from Schwann Cells that grow into a mass on the vestibular nerve, often leading to progressive hearing loss and vertigo. It is usually unilateral. Bilateral cases are a concern for hereditary diseases. It is usually a benign tumor, thus there is no concern for metastasis.
- Mechanism: a slow growth of cells that will eventually become a large mass. This causes a mass effect, compressing its local environment, including the

cranial nerve of hearing and balance.
- Clinical Features: Early on patients may present with unilateral sensorineural hearing loss, tinnitus, and vertigo. Later on, late manifestations can include facial weakness, numbness, and headaches.
- Clinical Insight: Early diagnosis is crucial for effective management and preservation of hearing.

Stroke:

- Description: an acute neurologic condition that is caused by lack of blood flow to the brain. This can be caused by a blood vessel that ruptures or a blood vessel that clots. Depending on the

location of the blood vessel, a stroke can cause vertigo, specifically central vertigo.
- Connection to Vertigo: vertigo can be a symptom of certain strokes, especially those affecting the brainstem or cerebellum. When vertigo occurs due to the pathologic conditions in the brain, this is considered **central vertigo**. Compared to peripheral vertigo, central vertigo is a medical emergency.
- Clinical Features: patients may present with vertigo, but most often patients will present with double vision (diplopia), trouble speaking (dysarthria), facial drooping, and trouble swallowing (dysphagia).

- Critical Aspect: prompt medical attention is essential for differentiating stroke-related vertigo from other causes.

Medications:

- Drug-Induced Vertigo: Certain medications can contribute to vertigo as a side effect.
- Caution: Consultation with a healthcare provider is necessary to evaluate medication-related vertigo and explore alternative options.

Head Trauma:

- Traumatic Vertigo: Head injuries can disrupt the inner ear or vestibular system, resulting in

persistent vertigo. Benign paroxysmal positional vertigo can often be associated with a head trauma as well.
- Clinical Guidance: Comprehensive evaluation following head trauma is crucial for appropriate intervention.

In conclusion, a thorough understanding of the diverse causes of vertigo is pivotal for healthcare professionals and individuals alike. The complexity of these conditions underscores the importance of seeking expert medical guidance for accurate diagnosis and tailored treatment plans. By delving into the specifics of each cause, this chapter aims to empower readers with knowledge that facilitates informed discussions with healthcare providers, fostering optimal care and improved outcomes for those grappling with vertigo.

Chapter 5

Recognizing Critical Signs: When to Seek Urgent Medical Attention for Vertigo

Understanding when to seek medical care for vertigo is crucial in ensuring timely intervention and appropriate treatment. This chapter explores the guidelines provided by reputable sources, such as the Mayo Clinic, to help individuals identify situations warranting emergency medical attention when experiencing vertigo.

According to the Mayo Clinic, individuals with vertigo should promptly seek emergency medical treatment if they encounter new, severe dizziness or vertigo, particularly if accompanied by any of the following alarming symptoms:

Sudden Severe Headaches:

- Significance: Sudden and intense headaches could be indicative of various underlying medical conditions, including those affecting the brain.
- If you think this the "worst headache of your life," then urgently go to the nearest emergency department

Cardiovascular Symptoms:

- Manifestations: Chest pain, difficulty breathing, and symptoms such as numbness or paralysis of arms or legs may suggest cardiovascular issues requiring immediate attention.

Neurological Abnormalities:

- Indicators: Fainting, double vision, rapid or irregular heartbeat, confusion, slurred speech, stumbling, or difficulty walking could signify neurological complications.

Gastrointestinal Distress:

- Concerns: Ongoing vomiting, especially when persistent, may lead to dehydration and demands assessment for potential serious underlying causes.

Seizures:

- Implications: The occurrence of seizures demands immediate medical evaluation to identify and address their root causes.

Sensory Changes:

- Red Flags: A sudden change in hearing, facial numbness or weakness may signal neurological or sensory system involvement.

(Mayo Clinic Guidelines)

Additional Considerations:

Apart from the Mayo Clinic guidelines, it is essential to recognize that vertigo can sometimes be a symptom of serious underlying medical conditions. Seeking medical care is warranted in the following situations:

Recurrent or Prolonged Episodes:

- Explanation: Frequent or extended bouts of vertigo may indicate chronic conditions that necessitate medical evaluation.

Vertigo Following Head Trauma:
- Rationale: If vertigo occurs after a head injury, it is crucial to rule out potential vestibular or neurological damage.

New-Onset Vertigo in Older Adults:
- Justification: Especially in older individuals, new-onset vertigo may be associated with cardiovascular or neurological concerns, requiring thorough assessment.

Vertigo with Coexisting Medical Conditions:

- Consideration: Individuals with pre-existing medical conditions, such as heart disease or diabetes, should promptly seek medical care if experiencing vertigo to prevent complications.

Recognizing the critical signs that warrant urgent medical attention for vertigo is paramount for individuals experiencing these symptoms. By adhering to established guidelines and considering additional factors, such as recurrent episodes or pre-existing medical conditions, individuals can make informed decisions about seeking timely medical care. This approach facilitates early intervention, accurate diagnosis, and appropriate management, ultimately contributing to better outcomes and improved overall health.

Chapter 6

The Comprehensive Medical History in Vertigo Assessment

Medical history is a cornerstone in the evaluation of patients experiencing vertigo. When discussing your symptoms with a healthcare provider, precision and thoroughness are paramount. This chapter delves into the intricacies of obtaining a comprehensive medical history, guiding patients and providers alike toward a more nuanced understanding of the potential causes of vertigo.

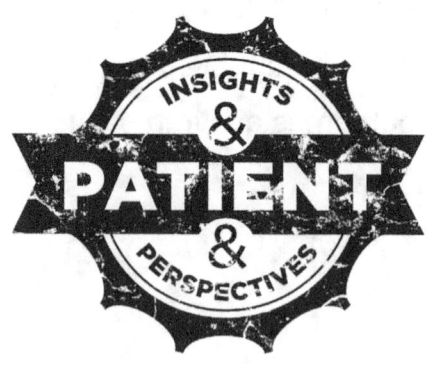 The following **medical history**

questions are **not** designed to be a comprehensive listing, however positive responses to any of the questions may provide clues as to the cause of a patient's vertigo. Take some time and look through the questions. Feel free to check boxes as you go. If you decide to visit a health care provider for your vertigo, your answers (both negative and affirmative) will be very helpful in determining a diagnosis. In the course of our careers, we have learned to simply ask open ended questions of patients with vertigo, and let them fill in the details, rather than asking simple yes or no questions. If we allow the vertigo patient to express what their symptoms are in their own words, more often than not, the patient will let us know if they have true vertigo and point us to a likely cause of their vertigo, even prior to the physical examination.

Essential Components of the Medical History:

<u>Current Symptoms and Previous Episodes:</u>
- ☐ Provide detailed information about the nature and duration of your current vertigo symptoms.
- ☐ Report any previous episodes of vertigo, specifying their frequency and intensity.

<u>Ear and Hearing History:</u>
- ☐ Any history of ear surgery, drainage or pain.
- ☐ Document recent changes in hearing, ear fullness, or pressure.
- ☐ Note any tinnitus, describing its characteristics such as pitch, quality, and association with pulse.

<u>Vertigo Symptoms:</u>

- ☐ Specify the duration of vertigo episodes and whether they are brief or continuous.
- ☐ Describe the sensation during an episode, including the perception of spinning, floating, falling, or being pushed in a particular direction.
- ☐ Explore how positional changes may exacerbate vertigo.

Falls and Assistive Devices:

- ☐ Report any falls or injuries related to vertigo.
- ☐ Indicate if assistive devices like canes or walkers are required for stability.

Associated Symptoms:

- ☐ Note any associated symptoms, such as blurred or double vision,

- weakness, or numbness in arms, legs, or face.
- ☐ Report any history of head trauma, neck injury, or cervical spine arthritis.

Medication History:

- ☐ List all current medications and recent changes in dosages.
- ☐ Mention any new medications or alterations in the weeks leading up to the onset of vertigo.

Hormonal and Pregnancy History:

- ☐ Document the use of hormonal supplements or contraceptives, especially those containing estrogen.
- ☐ Inquire about pregnancy or recent pregnancies.

Dietary and Allergy Considerations:

- ☐ Explore recent changes in diet, including processed foods or any high-sodium products.
- ☐ Inquire about allergies and medications taken for allergies.

Social and Mental Health:

- ☐ Assess mental health conditions, including depression, anxiety, or panic attacks.
- ☐ Inquire about recent life stressors and medications for mental health.

Diabetes and Blood Sugar Control:

- ☐ If applicable, report any numbness in the feet or toes.
- ☐ Evaluate the control of blood sugars and the use of diabetes medications.

The Significance of a Comprehensive Medical History:

The questions presented here offer a framework for gathering information that may provide crucial clues to the cause of vertigo. Positive responses to any questions can guide healthcare providers in formulating a diagnosis and developing an appropriate treatment plan. It is important to consider these aspects as interconnected, as vertigo can result from a combination of factors.

Clinical Tip: Open-ended questions that allow patients to articulate their symptoms in their own words often yield valuable insights. Patients sharing their experiences may lead to early identification of potential causes before a formal examination.

In conclusion, medical history is a dynamic tool that aids in unraveling the complexities of vertigo. Whether seeking care or providing care, the collaboration between patients and healthcare providers ensures a more accurate diagnosis and effective management of vertigo.

Chapter 7

Physical Examination for Patients with Vertigo

Vertigo is a sensation of spinning or dizziness that can be unsettling and disorienting for patients. Conducting a thorough physical examination is crucial for diagnosing the underlying cause of vertigo and planning an effective treatment strategy. This chapter will guide you through the key components of a physical examination for patients presenting with vertigo, providing a comprehensive approach to evaluating this complex symptom.

A detailed physical examination should include an assessment of the patient's general appearance, vital signs, and specific maneuvers to identify the cause of vertigo.

General Appearance and Vital Signs

Appearance: Note if the patient appears anxious or unsteady.

Vital Signs: Measure blood pressure, heart rate, and temperature. Orthostatic vital signs can help identify postural hypotension, a potential cause of dizziness.

Neurological Examination

A focused neurological examination is crucial to rule out central causes of vertigo.

Cranial Nerve Examination:

Assess all cranial nerves, with particular attention to the following:

Cranial Nerve **II** (Optic): Visual acuity and field testing.

Cranial Nerve **III, IV, VI** (Oculomotor, Trochlear, Abducens): Eye movements to look for nystagmus (involuntary eye movement) and ocular alignment.

Cranial Nerve **VIII** (Vestibulocochlear): Hearing tests and balance assessment.

Cranial Nerve **VII** (Facial): if facial weakness is noted on either or both sides, ear disease may contribute to vertigo.

2. Motor System Examination: Check muscle strength, tone, and coordination.

3. Sensory System Examination: Test for sensation changes, particularly proprioception (ability to feel the floor) and vibration sense.

4. Gait and Balance: Observe the patient's gait for any abnormalities and perform specific balance tests.

Otologic (Ear) Examination:

In patients presenting with vertigo, a detailed otologic (ear) examination is crucial to identify or rule out conditions affecting the middle and inner ears, which are common causes of vertigo. Here are the key components and findings to focus on during the otologic examination:

Otoscopic Examination

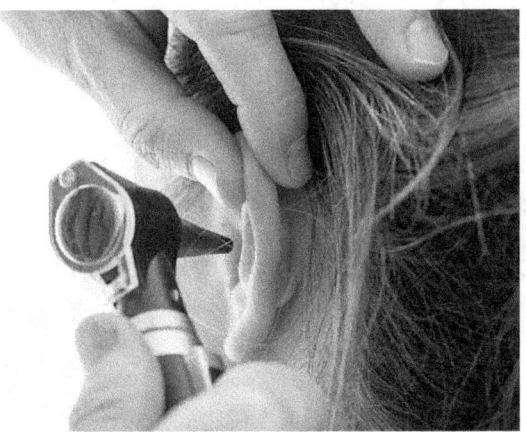

External Ear

Inspect the external ear: Look for any signs of deformities, lesions, or discharge that could indicate infection or other pathologies.

Palpate the auricle and tragus: Assess for tenderness, which might suggest otitis externa (outer ear infection).

Ear Canal and Tympanic Membrane

Examine the ear canal: Check for cerumen (wax) impaction, foreign bodies, or signs of infection or inflammation.

Inspect the tympanic membrane: Assess for color, position, integrity, and presence of fluid behind the membrane.

Normal Tympanic Membrane: Pearly gray and translucent.

Abnormal Findings:
- Redness or Bulging: Indicates acute otitis media.

- Retraction: Suggests Eustachian tube dysfunction.

- Perforation: Presence of a hole or rupture.

- Fluid Level or Bubbles: Indicates middle ear effusion, possibly related to serous otitis media.

- Redness or mass behind tympanic membrane: May indicate a tumor.

In Office Hearing Assessment

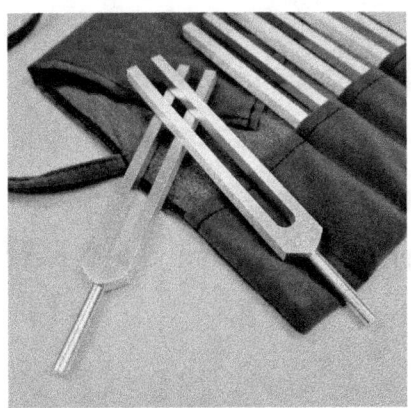

Tuning Fork Tests

Weber Test:

 - Strike the tuning fork and place it on the midline of the forehead.

 - Ask the patient where they hear the sound (left ear, right ear, or both equally).

 - Interpretation:

   - Normal: Sound is heard equally in both ears.

   - Conductive Hearing Loss: Sound is heard louder in the affected ear.

   - Sensorineural Hearing Loss: Sound is heard louder in the unaffected ear.

Rinne Test:

 - Strike the tuning fork and place it on the mastoid process (bone) behind the ear.

 - Ask the patient to indicate when the sound is no longer heard, then move the tuning fork near the ear canal.

 - Interpretation:

- Normal (Positive Rinne): Air conduction is heard louder than bone conduction.
- Conductive Hearing Loss (Negative Rinne): Bone conduction is heard louder than air conduction.
- Sensorineural Hearing Loss: Both air and bone conduction are reduced, but air conduction is still heard longer.

Cardiovascular Examination

Since vertigo can also be related to cardiovascular issues, a thorough cardiovascular assessment is necessary.

Heart Auscultation: Listen for abnormal heart sounds or murmurs.

Carotid Bruits: Check for bruits (noisy blood flow) indicating carotid artery stenosis.

Peripheral Pulses: Assess for peripheral artery disease.

Physical Examination Clues:

While the majority of patients with vertigo may exhibit a normal physical examination, subtle findings can provide valuable clues. These include:

Nystagmus:
- Definition: Involuntary twitching or rotation of the eyes, often triggered by positional changes.
- Significance: Can offer insights into the origin of vertigo.

Numbness or Weakness:
- In the arms, legs, or face may suggest neurological involvement.

Ear Infection Evidence:
- Especially relevant in children, as fluid behind the eardrum can be a common cause of vertigo.

Middle Ear Tumors:
- Detection of tumors like "glomus" in the region between the eardrum and inner ear.

Neurological Testing:
- Romberg test: Assessing stability when standing with arms outstretched and eyes closed.
- Finger-to-nose test: Evaluating cerebellar function.
- Unterberger (Fakuda's Stepping) test: Marching in place with eyes closed to reveal inner ear imbalances.

Conducting a meticulous physical examination is essential for accurately diagnosing the cause of vertigo. By following the steps outlined in this chapter, healthcare providers can differentiate between various etiologies and develop a targeted treatment plan. Remember, the key to effective management of vertigo lies in a thorough understanding of the patient's symptoms and a systematic approach to examination.

Chapter 8

Understanding Vertigo Tests: A Comprehensive Guide for Patients

When it comes to identifying the underlying causes of vertigo, several tests play a crucial role in guiding healthcare professionals toward accurate diagnoses and tailored treatments. Before delving into these tests, it's essential to emphasize the significance of a thorough medical history and physical examination, as they lay the foundation for targeted investigations.

Imaging studies for Vertigo:

Imaging studies are vital tools used by doctors to understand and treat vertigo. These tests help identify any structural issues or abnormalities in the body that could be causing the vertigo symptoms. While most vertigo cases are linked to harmless conditions like vestibular migraine or benign paroxysmal positional vertigo (BPPV), imaging is crucial to rule out more serious problems like vestibular schwannoma (a tumor), stroke, or other brain disorders.

Doctors decide to use imaging based on various factors such as age, medical history, severity of symptoms, and any existing neurological problems. They often recommend imaging for vertigo patients with unusual symptoms, sudden onset of symptoms, symptoms that don't improve with treatment, or a history of head injuries. People with certain health conditions like high blood pressure, diabetes, or cancer may also need imaging to check for potential issues in the brain.

Different types of imaging tests can be used, including magnetic resonance imaging (MRI) and computed tomography (CT) scans. MRI is usually preferred because it gives detailed images of the brain and inner ear structures. It can reveal problems like tumors, bleeding in the brain, or abnormal blood vessels that might be causing vertigo. CT scans are sometimes used if MRI isn't possible, and are excellent for showing boney defects, but they aren't as good at showing certain soft tissue causes such as small tumors.

The results of these imaging tests can be crucial for diagnosis and treatment. They might show that there are no serious problems, which can be reassuring for the patient and help confirm a diagnosis of a harmless condition. However, if a problem is found, it could mean further treatment is needed. For instance, finding a tumor might mean surgery or other treatments are necessary. Overall, imaging tests are essential for doctors to understand what's causing vertigo and how to best help patients manage it.

Audiometric and Balance Testing:

This test is vital for establishing a diagnosis, especially when vertigo is accompanied by:

- Hearing loss in one or both ears.
- Tinnitus (ringing in the ears).
- Sensations of ear pressure or plugging.
- History of deafness or prior ear surgery.

A standard complete audiogram is a common diagnostic test used to assess a person's hearing ability across different frequencies and volumes. Here's what typically happens during the test:

Preparation:

You'll be seated in a soundproof booth or room to minimize background noise interference.

The audiologist will explain the procedure and answer any questions you may have.

Tone Testing:

You'll wear headphones or earphones connected to an audiometer, a machine that generates sounds at various frequencies and volumes. You'll be asked to indicate each time you hear a sound by pressing a button or raising your hand.

Air Conduction Testing: The audiologist will present tones at different frequencies (pitch) and volumes (loudness) to each ear separately. They start with low frequencies and gradually increase to higher ones. This helps determine the softest sounds you can hear across the entire frequency range.

Bone Conduction Testing: In some cases, bone conduction testing may be performed. A bone oscillator is placed behind the ear to bypass the outer and middle ear and directly stimulate the inner ear. This helps determine if hearing loss is due to problems in the outer or middle ear (conductive hearing loss) or the inner ear (sensorineural hearing loss).

Speech Testing: You may also undergo speech testing, where you listen to recorded speech at different volumes to assess your ability to understand spoken words.

Results: The audiologist will plot your responses on a graph called an audiogram, which shows your hearing thresholds (the softest sounds you can hear) at different frequencies. The audiogram helps identify the type, degree, and configuration of any hearing loss. Results are typically discussed with you after the test, and recommendations for further evaluation or treatment, such as hearing aids or medical intervention, may be provided if necessary.

Overall, a standard complete audiogram provides valuable information about your hearing health and helps audiologists tailor treatment plans to address any hearing or vestibular difficulties you may be experiencing.

Differences in hearing between the ears can provide crucial clues. If you've undergone previous hearing tests, bringing copies to your healthcare provider can aid in tracking changes over time. For instance, a sudden hearing loss audiogram (like the one mentioned in the book) due to a tumor on the acoustic nerve could be indicative of specific conditions.

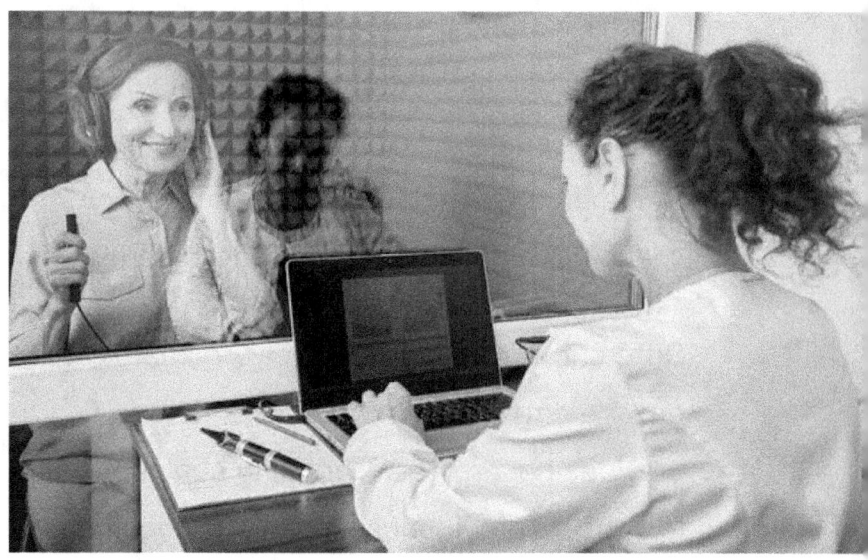

Patient undergoing audiometric testing in a sound booth

Tympanograms:

This test measures the pressure of the middle ear (behind the eardrum). Abnormal pressures (negative or positive) may contribute to vertigo, especially in children with a history of middle ear infections. Approximately 66% of children with chronic middle ear fluid may exhibit abnormalities on inner ear and balance testing.

Tympanograms play a crucial role in assessing the health of the middle ear, which can have implications for individuals experiencing vertigo. A tympanogram is a simple and painless test used to evaluate the function of the eardrum and the middle ear space behind it. During the test, a soft rubber tip is placed in the ear canal, and air pressure is gently changed to measure how well the eardrum responds. Tympanograms provide valuable information about the mobility and pressure of the middle ear, helping healthcare providers identify conditions that may contribute to vertigo symptoms.

Understanding the importance of tympanograms for patients with vertigo involves recognizing that abnormalities in middle ear function can affect vestibular function and contribute to vertigo. For example, conditions such as otitis media (middle ear infection), eustachian tube dysfunction, or tympanic membrane perforation can disrupt the delicate balance of pressure within the middle ear, leading to vertigo or dizziness. Tympanograms help detect these abnormalities by revealing characteristic patterns that indicate issues such as fluid accumulation, impaired mobility of the eardrum, or abnormal pressure equalization.

Abnormal tympanogram results can provide valuable insights into the underlying causes of vertigo and guide appropriate management strategies. For instance, if tympanograms indicate the presence of middle ear fluid (effusion), healthcare providers may recommend treatment with antibiotics or decongestants to address any underlying infection or inflammation. Similarly, if tympanograms reveal eustachian tube dysfunction or other structural abnormalities, interventions such as ear tube placement or surgical repair may be considered to restore middle ear function and alleviate vertigo symptoms. By recognizing the significance of tympanograms in the evaluation of vertigo, individuals can work collaboratively with their healthcare providers to address middle ear issues and optimize vestibular health.

The HINT Test: A Valuable Tool in Diagnosing Vertigo

The Head-Impulse, Nystagmus, Test of Skew (HINT) is a clinical test designed to aid in the diagnosis of vestibular disorders, particularly those causing vertigo. This simple yet effective test can provide valuable insights into the function of the vestibular system, helping clinicians differentiate between peripheral and central causes of vertigo.

How Does the HINT Test Work?

The HINT test consists of three components:

Head Impulse Test (HIT): In this part of the test, the clinician asks the patient to fixate on a target while the head is briskly rotated to one side. The clinician then observes the patient's eyes for any corrective saccades, which are rapid, involuntary eye movements that indicate a vestibular deficit.

Nystagmus Examination: The clinician examines the patient for nystagmus, which is an involuntary rhythmic oscillation of the eyes. Different patterns of nystagmus can indicate peripheral or central vestibular dysfunction.

Test of Skew: The clinician assesses for skew deviation, which is a vertical misalignment of the eyes that can occur in central vestibular disorders.

Clinical Significance of the HINT Test

The HINT test is particularly useful in differentiating between peripheral and central causes of vertigo. Peripheral vestibular disorders, such as benign paroxysmal positional vertigo (BPPV), vestibular neuritis, and Meniere's disease, typically result in abnormal HIT findings with corrective saccades and characteristic patterns of nystagmus. In contrast, central vestibular disorders, such as vestibular migraine, cerebellar infarction, and multiple sclerosis, may present with normal HIT but abnormal findings on other components of the test, such as nystagmus or skew deviation.

Advantages of the HINT Test

The HINT test offers several advantages in the evaluation of vertigo:

>Rapid and Easy to Perform: The test can be quickly administered at the bedside,

making it a practical tool in the clinical setting.

High Sensitivity and Specificity: The HINT test has been shown to have high sensitivity and specificity for detecting vestibular dysfunction, aiding in accurate diagnosis.

Helps Guide Management: The results of the HINT test can help clinicians determine the appropriate management strategy for patients with vertigo, whether it be vestibular rehabilitation, pharmacotherapy, or further diagnostic evaluation.

In conclusion, the HINT test is a valuable clinical tool in the evaluation of vertigo, providing important information about the function of the vestibular system and aiding in the differentiation of peripheral and central causes of vertigo. Its simplicity, ease of administration, and clinical utility make it a valuable addition to the diagnostic armamentarium for vestibular disorders.

ENG

If you've been experiencing vertigo, you might have heard about ENG testing. ENG, or electronystagmography, is a diagnostic test used to evaluate dizziness and balance problems. It's a non-invasive procedure that helps doctors understand what might be causing your symptoms. During the test, electrodes are placed around your eyes to monitor eye movements while you undergo a series of positional changes and visual stimuli. These eye movements are crucial indicators of inner ear function and can reveal issues such as vestibular dysfunction or abnormalities in the vestibular system.

Understanding the importance of ENG testing can help you get the right diagnosis and treatment for your vertigo. Vertigo can significantly impact your quality of life, affecting your ability to work, drive, or even perform simple daily tasks. By pinpointing the underlying cause of your vertigo through ENG testing, doctors can tailor a treatment plan that addresses your specific condition. Whether it's benign paroxysmal positional vertigo (BPPV), Meniere's disease, or another vestibular disorder, timely diagnosis is key to managing symptoms effectively and improving your overall well-being.

After undergoing ENG testing, you'll receive results that provide valuable insights into your vestibular function. These results help your healthcare provider determine the most appropriate course of action for managing your vertigo. Depending on the findings, treatment options may include vestibular rehabilitation exercises, medication, or in some cases, surgical intervention. ENG testing empowers both patients and healthcare professionals by offering objective data to guide treatment decisions and optimize outcomes, ultimately helping individuals regain their balance and conquer vertigo's challenges.

Posturography

Vestibular posturography testing is a crucial tool in the diagnosis and management of vertigo and balance disorders. This specialized test assesses your body's ability to maintain balance by measuring your postural stability in various conditions. During the test, you'll stand on a force platform while wearing a safety harness, and your movements will be monitored as the platform tilts or moves in different directions. By analyzing your responses to these controlled stimuli, healthcare providers can evaluate the function of your vestibular system, which plays a central role in maintaining balance and spatial orientation.

Understanding the importance of vestibular posturography testing can help individuals struggling with vertigo gain clarity about their condition and receive targeted treatment. Vertigo and balance problems can stem from a wide range of underlying issues, including inner ear disorders, neurological conditions, or musculoskeletal impairments. By undergoing vestibular posturography testing, patients can uncover the root cause of their symptoms and work with their healthcare team to develop personalized treatment plans. This comprehensive approach not only addresses immediate concerns but also helps prevent falls and improve overall quality of life.

Upon completion of vestibular posturography testing, individuals receive detailed results that provide valuable insights into their balance function and vestibular health. These results help guide treatment decisions and monitor progress over time. Depending on the findings, treatment strategies may include vestibular rehabilitation exercises, lifestyle modifications, or referrals to other specialists for further evaluation. By leveraging the information gleaned from vestibular posturography testing, patients can take proactive steps towards managing their vertigo and regaining confidence in their ability to navigate the world safely.

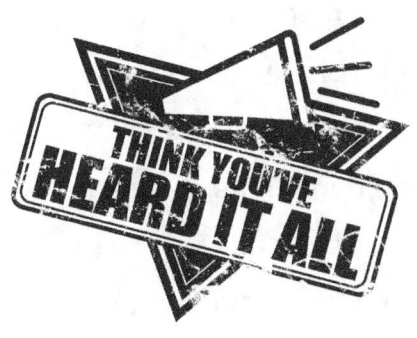

Spinning chair vestibular testing is a specialized diagnostic procedure used to assess the function of the vestibular system, which is responsible for balance and spatial orientation. During the test, you'll be comfortably seated in a chair that can rotate in different directions while wearing a set of goggles equipped with cameras to track eye movements. The chair will gradually rotate at varying speeds, stimulating your vestibular system and eliciting specific eye movements called nystagmus. By analyzing these eye movements and your subjective sensations of dizziness or vertigo, healthcare providers can gain valuable insights into the health of your inner ear and vestibular function.

Understanding the importance of spinning chair vestibular testing can provide individuals experiencing vertigo with clarity and direction in managing their symptoms. Vertigo can stem from various underlying conditions, including disorders of the inner ear such as Meniere's disease or vestibular neuritis. By undergoing spinning chair vestibular testing, patients can pinpoint the specific nature of their vestibular dysfunction and work with their healthcare team to tailor treatment plans accordingly. Whether it involves medication, vestibular rehabilitation exercises, or other interventions, the insights gleaned from this test can help individuals regain their balance and alleviate the disruptive effects of vertigo on their daily lives.

Hallpike Tests

The Hallpike maneuver is a common diagnostic test used to assess and diagnose a type of vertigo called benign paroxysmal positional vertigo (BPPV). BPPV occurs when tiny calcium carbonate crystals in the inner ear become dislodged and float into one of the fluid-filled canals responsible for balance. This displacement can cause brief episodes of intense vertigo triggered by changes in head position. The Hallpike maneuver helps healthcare providers identify which ear is affected and which specific canal is involved.

During the Hallpike maneuver, you'll be seated upright on an examination table with your legs extended. The healthcare provider will then guide you into a specific lying position, typically with your head turned to one side and tilted slightly backward over the edge of the table. This position is maintained for a brief period, allowing any loose crystals to move within the affected canal. If BPPV is present, you may experience a brief, intense spinning sensation called vertigo, accompanied by characteristic eye movements known as nystagmus. The maneuver may be repeated on the opposite side to confirm the diagnosis and identify any additional affected canals.

Understanding the importance of the Hallpike maneuver can help individuals experiencing vertigo find relief and targeted treatment. BPPV is a common cause of vertigo, especially among older adults, and can significantly impact daily activities and quality of life. By accurately diagnosing BPPV through the Hallpike maneuver, healthcare providers can recommend specific maneuvers or exercises, such as the Epley maneuver or Brandt-Daroff exercises, to help reposition the displaced crystals and alleviate vertigo symptoms. Additionally, knowing the underlying cause of vertigo can provide reassurance and empower individuals to actively participate in their treatment plan. While the Hallpike maneuver itself may induce temporary vertigo, the information gained from the test is invaluable in guiding effective management strategies and improving overall well-being.

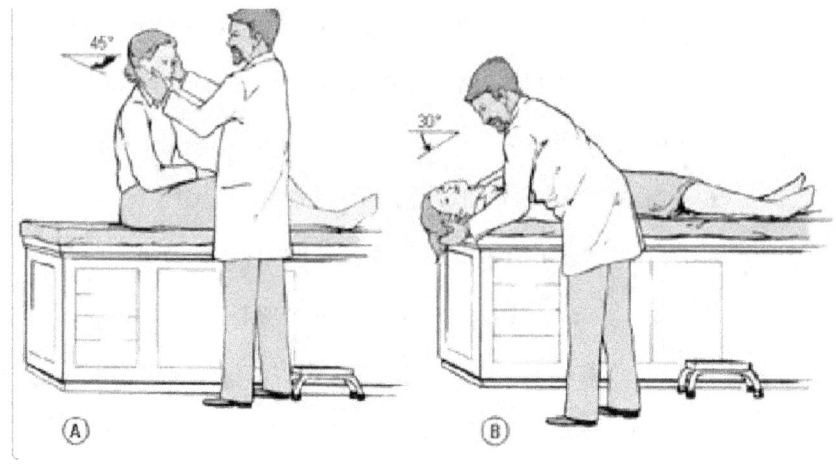

Hallpike Testing

Frenzel lenses

Frenzel lenses are a crucial tool used during vestibular testing to enhance the accuracy of the examination and provide valuable insights into the function of the vestibular system. These lenses are essentially magnifying glasses equipped with a light source, allowing healthcare providers to closely observe and record eye movements, particularly nystagmus, which is a key indicator of vestibular dysfunction. By wearing Frenzel lenses, any involuntary eye movements become more

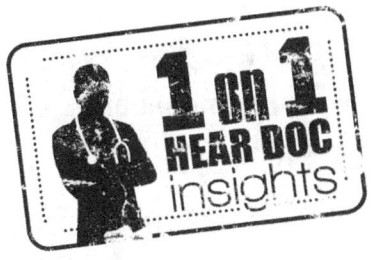

apparent and easier to analyze, aiding in the diagnosis of various vestibular disorders.

It's understandable that some individuals may feel apprehensive about wearing Frenzel lenses during vestibular testing, especially if they're already experiencing discomfort or dizziness. However, it's important to note that Frenzel lenses themselves do not cause or exacerbate vertigo symptoms. Instead, they serve as a diagnostic tool to help healthcare providers accurately assess vestibular function and identify the underlying cause of vertigo. While wearing Frenzel lenses, you may be asked to perform specific head movements or positional changes to elicit nystagmus, but rest assured that these maneuvers are conducted in a controlled and supervised environment.

Ultimately, Frenzel lenses play a crucial role in facilitating the accurate diagnosis and effective management of vestibular disorders, including vertigo. Rather than being feared, they should be seen as an essential component of the diagnostic process, helping to provide clarity and guidance in addressing vertigo symptoms. Trusting in the expertise of your healthcare provider and understanding the purpose of Frenzel lenses can help alleviate any concerns and pave the way for targeted treatment strategies to improve your vestibular health and overall well-being.

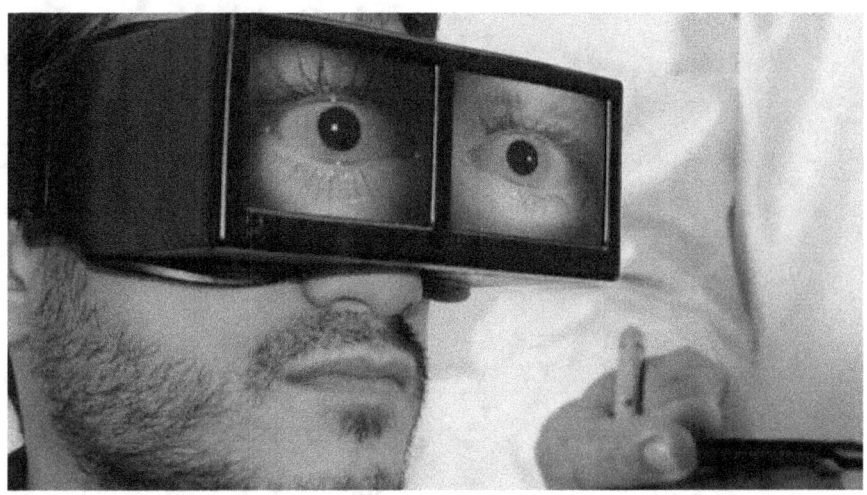

Patient Wearing **Frenzel Lenses** to Measure Eye Movements

Understanding the Testing Process:

Preparation:
- Familiarize yourself with your medical history, especially details related to hearing, ear surgeries, and prior hearing tests.

Communication:

- Discuss any associated symptoms like hearing loss, tinnitus, or ear pressure with your healthcare provider.

Collaboration:
- Work with your healthcare team to understand the implications of test results and how they contribute to the overall diagnosis.

Clinical Insight: The aforementioned tests collectively offer a comprehensive view of the factors contributing to vertigo. Regular monitoring through hearing tests, in particular, can be instrumental in tracking changes over time.

In conclusion, undergoing these tests, along with providing a detailed medical history, is an essential step in unraveling the mysteries of vertigo. Collaborating with your healthcare provider, asking questions, and staying informed about your test results empowers you to actively participate in your care journey.

Chapter 9

Understanding Ophthalmologic Causes of Vertigo

Vertigo, a sensation of spinning or dizziness, can be a distressing symptom with various underlying causes. While it is commonly associated with inner ear issues, ophthalmologic conditions can also contribute to vertigo. This chapter explores these causes, the diagnostic tests used to identify them, and the treatment and prevention strategies available.

Ophthalmologic Causes of Vertigo

Several ophthalmologic conditions can lead to vertigo:

a. Optic neuritis: Inflammation of the optic nerve, often associated with multiple sclerosis, can cause vertigo due to its impact on visual input and the vestibular system's function.

b. Retinal migraine: This condition involves temporary visual disturbances followed by a headache. It can lead to vertigo, likely due to its effects on the visual and vestibular systems.

c. Central serous chorioretinopathy (CSCR): CSCR is characterized by fluid buildup under the retina. Although rare, it can cause vertigo, possibly due to its impact on retinal function.

d. Macular degeneration: While primarily a cause of vision loss, advanced macular degeneration can affect balance and lead to a sensation of vertigo.

Diagnostic Tests for Ophthalmologic Causes of Vertigo

a. Visual acuity test: Evaluates how clearly each eye can see. Abnormalities may suggest optic nerve or retinal disorders.

b. Visual field test: Assesses peripheral vision, crucial for detecting abnormalities related to optic nerve or retinal issues.

c. Fundoscopic exam: Examines the back of the eye for signs of inflammation, fluid accumulation, or other abnormalities.

d. Optical coherence tomography (OCT): Provides detailed images of the retina, helping diagnose conditions like CSCR and macular degeneration.

Treatment and Prevention

a. Treatment: Management of ophthalmologic causes of vertigo often focuses on treating the underlying eye condition. This may involve medications, such as corticosteroids for optic neuritis, or anti-VEGF drugs for CSCR.

b. Prevention: Regular eye exams are essential for early detection and management of ophthalmologic conditions that can lead to vertigo. Maintaining overall eye health through a balanced diet, regular exercise, and protective eyewear can also help prevent these issues.

While vertigo is commonly linked to inner ear problems, ophthalmologic causes should also be considered, especially when accompanied by visual disturbances. Early diagnosis and management of these conditions are crucial for preventing complications and improving quality of life.

Chapter 10

Navigating Treatment Options for Dizziness and Vertigo

Experiencing dizziness and vertigo can be disconcerting, affecting one's daily life and overall well-being. Fortunately, there are various treatment options available to alleviate these symptoms and restore a sense of balance. In this chapter, we will explore both medical and lifestyle interventions that can be beneficial for individuals grappling with dizziness and vertigo.

Medical Interventions:

Vestibular Rehabilitation Therapy (VRT):

- Description: VRT is a specialized form of physical therapy designed to improve vestibular

function and reduce symptoms of dizziness and imbalance.
- How It Works: Trained therapists guide individuals through exercises that stimulate the vestibular system, enhancing its ability to coordinate with vision and proprioception.

Medications:

- Antihistamines: Drugs like meclizine can alleviate symptoms by reducing inner ear excitability.
- Benzodiazepines: Medications like diazepam may be prescribed to alleviate vertigo symptoms.

Canalith Repositioning Procedures:

- Description: Techniques like the Epley maneuver are effective for benign paroxysmal positional

vertigo (BPPV), where displaced calcium crystals are repositioned in the inner ear.
- Effectiveness: High success rates are reported for BPPV cases treated with canalith repositioning procedures.

Lifestyle and Home Remedies:

Stay Hydrated:
- Rationale: Dehydration can exacerbate dizziness, so it's crucial to maintain adequate fluid intake.
- Tip: Carry a reusable water bottle to ensure regular hydration throughout the day.

Balanced Diet:
- Importance: Nutrient deficiencies can contribute to dizziness.

- Recommendation: Consume a well-balanced diet rich in vitamins and minerals, particularly B-complex vitamins.

Manage Stress:
- Stress Connection: Anxiety and stress can amplify vertigo symptoms.
- Techniques: Practice relaxation methods such as deep breathing, meditation, or yoga to manage stress levels.

Physical Activity:
- Benefits: Engaging in regular, moderate exercise can enhance overall well-being and reduce the frequency and severity of vertigo episodes.

Sleep Hygiene:
- Impact: Poor sleep can worsen dizziness and imbalance.
- Advice: Establish a consistent sleep routine and create a comfortable sleep environment.

The journey to alleviate dizziness and vertigo involves a combination of medical interventions and lifestyle adjustments. Seeking professional guidance is essential to determine the most suitable treatment plan for individual cases. By incorporating vestibular rehabilitation, appropriate medications, and adopting healthy lifestyle habits, individuals can take meaningful steps towards managing their symptoms and regaining control over their lives. Remember, persistence and collaboration with healthcare professionals are key elements in achieving success on the path to recovery.

Chapter 11

Physical Therapy for Vertigo

Vestibular rehabilitation therapy (VRT) has emerged as a highly effective treatment approach for individuals suffering from vertigo and other vestibular disorders. VRT is a specialized form of physical therapy designed to address symptoms such as dizziness, imbalance, and vertigo by promoting central nervous system compensation for vestibular dysfunction. This form of therapy is tailored to each individual's specific symptoms, functional limitations, and underlying vestibular condition, making it a personalized and targeted approach to rehabilitation.

The indications for VRT are broad, encompassing various vestibular disorders that result in vertigo or balance disturbances. Common conditions treated with VRT include benign paroxysmal positional vertigo (BPPV), vestibular neuritis, labyrinthitis, Meniere's disease, and vestibular hypofunction. Indications for VRT may include persistent or recurrent vertigo, imbalance, unsteadiness, motion sensitivity, difficulty walking or performing daily activities, and a history of falls related to vestibular dysfunction. Additionally, VRT may be recommended as a component of comprehensive management for individuals undergoing surgical procedures affecting the vestibular system or experiencing vestibular symptoms following head trauma.

The results of VRT in vertigo patients are often remarkable, with many individuals experiencing significant improvements in symptoms and functional abilities. VRT aims to promote vestibular compensation, which refers to the brain's ability to adapt and adjust to vestibular dysfunction by relying on alternative sensory inputs and neural pathways. Through a series of exercises and maneuvers, VRT helps recalibrate the vestibular system, enhance balance control, improve gaze stability, and reduce symptoms of dizziness and vertigo. The specific exercises prescribed in VRT may include habituation exercises, gaze stabilization exercises, balance training, and canalith repositioning maneuvers, among others. These exercises are typically performed under the guidance of a trained physical therapist and can be customized to accommodate individual progress and goals.

Research has consistently demonstrated the effectiveness of VRT in reducing symptoms and improving functional outcomes for vertigo patients. Studies have shown that VRT can lead to significant reductions in dizziness severity, frequency of vertigo episodes, and postural instability, as well as improvements in overall quality of life and participation in daily activities. Furthermore, VRT has been found to decrease the risk of falls and enhance functional independence, allowing individuals to regain confidence and resume their normal activities with greater ease. Overall, VRT offers a safe, non-invasive, and evidence-based approach to managing vertigo and vestibular disorders, empowering individuals to achieve meaningful improvements in their vestibular function and quality of life.

Chapter 12

Dietary Treatments for Vertigo

Vertigo can be a challenging condition to manage. While medical interventions and physical therapy are commonly used treatments, dietary modifications can also play a role in alleviating symptoms and improving quality of life for individuals with vertigo. This guide explores the dietary factors that can impact vertigo and provides practical tips for incorporating dietary treatments into your daily routine.

Understanding the Role of Diet in Vertigo

Diet can influence vertigo through several mechanisms. Certain foods and beverages can affect blood flow, fluid balance, and neurotransmitter levels in the inner ear and brain, all of which are important for maintaining balance and equilibrium. By making mindful choices about what you eat and drink, you can potentially reduce the frequency and severity of vertigo episodes.

Foods and Beverages to Avoid

Certain foods and beverages may trigger or exacerbate vertigo symptoms. These include:

- High-sodium foods: Excessive sodium intake can lead to fluid

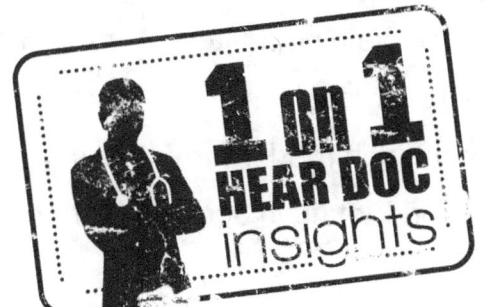

retention, which may increase pressure in the inner ear and worsen vertigo. Limiting sodium intake to less than 2,300 mg per day (or 1,500 mg per day for those with hypertension) is recommended. Even vegetables like celery are fairly high in natural sodium!
- Caffeine: Caffeine can stimulate the central nervous system and may increase anxiety and worsen vertigo symptoms in some individuals. Limiting or avoiding caffeinated beverages like coffee, tea, and soda may be beneficial.
- Alcohol: Alcohol can affect the central nervous system and disrupt the balance of fluids in the inner ear, potentially triggering vertigo. Limiting alcohol intake or avoiding it altogether may help manage symptoms.
- Tyramine-rich foods: Tyramine is a compound found in aged and fermented

foods that can trigger migraine headaches, which are often associated with vertigo. Foods high in tyramine include aged cheeses, cured meats, and certain fermented foods.
- Artificial sweeteners: Some studies suggest that artificial sweeteners like aspartame may trigger vertigo in some individuals. Avoiding foods and beverages containing these sweeteners may be beneficial.

Foods and Beverages That May Help

Certain foods and beverages may have a positive impact on vertigo symptoms. These include:

- Hydrating foods: Staying hydrated is important for maintaining fluid balance in the body, which can help reduce vertigo symptoms. Eating water-rich

foods like fruits and vegetables can contribute to your daily fluid intake.
- Magnesium-rich foods: Magnesium is a mineral that plays a role in muscle relaxation and may help reduce the frequency and severity of vertigo episodes. Foods rich in magnesium include leafy greens, nuts, seeds, and whole grains.
- Ginger: Ginger has anti-inflammatory properties and may help reduce nausea associated with vertigo. Consuming ginger tea or adding fresh ginger to your meals may be beneficial.
- Omega-3 fatty acids: Omega-3 fatty acids have anti-inflammatory effects and may help improve blood flow to the inner ear. Foods rich in omega-3s include fatty fish like salmon, walnuts, and flaxseeds.

Practical Tips for Incorporating Dietary Treatments

- Keep a food diary: Keeping track of your diet and any associated vertigo symptoms can help you identify trigger foods and make informed dietary choices.
- Consult with a healthcare professional: If you are considering dietary changes to manage vertigo, it is important to consult with a healthcare professional, such as a dietitian or otolaryngologist, to ensure that your diet is balanced and meets your nutritional needs.
- Gradual changes: Making gradual changes to your diet can help you

identify which foods may be triggering your vertigo symptoms without drastically altering your eating habits.

While dietary treatments for vertigo are not a substitute for medical intervention, they can be a valuable adjunctive therapy for managing symptoms and improving quality of life. By making informed choices about what you eat and drink, you can potentially reduce the frequency and severity of vertigo episodes and enjoy a more balanced and fulfilling life.

Chapter 13

Medicinal Treatments for Vertigo: An Overview

Vertigo, characterized by a spinning sensation or dizziness, can significantly impact an individual's quality of life. While there are various causes of vertigo, several medicinal treatments can help alleviate symptoms and improve daily functioning for those affected. This guide explores the different types of medicinal treatments available for vertigo sufferers, along with their benefits, considerations, and potential side effects.

Medications for Vertigo

Medications are often used to manage vertigo symptoms, depending on the underlying cause. Some common medications used to treat vertigo include:

- Antihistamines: Antihistamines such as meclizine and dimenhydrinate are commonly used to reduce nausea and dizziness associated with vertigo. They work by blocking histamine receptors in the brain.
- Anti-nausea medications: Medications like promethazine or ondansetron may be prescribed to alleviate nausea and vomiting associated with vertigo.
- Benzodiazepines: Drugs like diazepam or lorazepam may be used to reduce anxiety and calm the nervous system, which can help alleviate vertigo symptoms.
- Anticholinergics: Scopolamine patches are sometimes used to reduce dizziness and nausea associated with vertigo.
- Vestibular suppressants: Medications like betahistine or cinnarizine may be

used to suppress the vestibular system, reducing vertigo symptoms.

Considerations for Medicinal Treatment

When considering medicinal treatments for vertigo, it is essential to consult with a healthcare professional to determine the most appropriate treatment plan. Factors to consider include:

- Underlying cause: The underlying cause of vertigo will influence the choice of medication. For example, if vertigo is caused by Meniere's disease, medications that reduce fluid buildup in the inner ear may be prescribed.
- Side effects: Medications used to treat vertigo can have side effects such as drowsiness, dry mouth, and blurred vision. It is important to discuss these

potential side effects with your healthcare provider.
- Interaction with other medications: Some medications used to treat vertigo can interact with other medications you may be taking. It is important to inform your healthcare provider about all medications you are currently taking.

Chapter 14:

Physical Therapy for Vertigo: Regain Your Balance and Confidence

Vertigo, characterized by a spinning sensation or dizziness, can be a debilitating condition that affects your quality of life. However, physical therapy can be a highly effective treatment option for many individuals suffering from vertigo. This guide explores the role of physical therapy in managing vertigo, the different techniques used, and how it can help you regain your balance and confidence.

Understanding Vertigo and Its Causes

Vertigo is often caused by problems in the inner ear or vestibular system, which is responsible for maintaining balance and spatial orientation. Conditions such as benign paroxysmal positional vertigo (BPPV), vestibular neuritis, and Meniere's disease can all lead to vertigo symptoms. Physical therapy aims to address these underlying issues and improve vestibular function.

How Physical Therapy Can Help

What to Expect During Physical Therapy

During your initial physical therapy session, your therapist will perform a thorough evaluation to assess your symptoms and determine the best course of treatment. They will then create a personalized treatment plan tailored to your specific needs and goals. Treatment sessions may include a combination of hands-on techniques, exercises, and education about vertigo and its management.

Benefits of Physical Therapy for Vertigo

Physical therapy can offer several benefits for individuals with vertigo, including:

- Reduced dizziness and vertigo symptoms: Many individuals experience a significant reduction in the frequency and severity of vertigo episodes after undergoing physical therapy.
- Improved balance and stability: Physical therapy can help improve balance and reduce the risk of falls, enhancing overall safety and mobility.
- Increased confidence: By improving balance and reducing dizziness, physical therapy can help you feel more confident in your daily activities.

Physical therapy is a highly effective treatment option for many individuals suffering from vertigo. By addressing underlying vestibular issues and improving balance and stability, physical therapy can help you regain your independence and quality of life. If you are experiencing vertigo symptoms, consider speaking with your healthcare provider about the benefits of physical therapy.

Chapter 15

Surgical Treatments for Vertigo: Exploring Your Options

Vertigo, a spinning sensation or dizziness, can be a debilitating condition that significantly impacts your quality of life. While many cases of vertigo can be managed with non-invasive treatments such as medications or physical therapy, some individuals may require surgical intervention to alleviate their symptoms. This guide explores surgical treatments for vertigo, including the procedures involved, their benefits, and what to expect.

Types of Surgical Treatments

There are several surgical procedures that may be used to treat vertigo, depending on the underlying cause and severity of the symptoms. Some common surgical treatments for vertigo include:

- Endolymphatic sac decompression: This procedure is used to treat Meniere's disease, a condition characterized by fluid buildup in the inner ear. During the surgery, the surgeon creates a small opening in the endolymphatic sac to drain excess fluid, relieving pressure and reducing vertigo symptoms.
- Intratympanic medications: This is a simple procedure where a steroid or ototoxic medication is injected through the tympanic membrane into the middle ear or applied through a tiny tube into the middle ear for relief of vertigo symptoms. It however can be accompanied by some degree of hearing loss.

- Vestibular nerve section: This procedure is used to treat vertigo caused by vestibular schwannoma, a benign tumor of the vestibular nerve. During the surgery, the surgeon cuts the vestibular nerve to eliminate vertigo symptoms. This procedure can lead to hearing loss in the affected ear.
- Labyrinthectomy: This procedure is used to treat severe, disabling vertigo that does not respond to other treatments. During the surgery, the surgeon removes part or all of the labyrinth, the part of the inner ear responsible for balance. This procedure can cause hearing loss in the affected ear.

Definition:

- A labyrinthectomy aims to remove the labyrinth, which consists of both bony structures

(the *bony labyrinth*) and soft tissues (the *membranous labyrinth*).
  - The labyrinth plays a crucial role in both hearing and balance.
- Canal plugging (occlusion): This procedure is used to treat benign paroxysmal positional vertigo (BPPV), a condition caused by loose calcium crystals in the inner ear. During the surgery, the surgeon plugs the affected semicircular canal to prevent the fluid from moving and causing vertigo.

Benefits of Surgical Treatments

Surgical treatments for vertigo can offer several benefits, including:

- Reduced vertigo symptoms: Surgical treatments can help alleviate vertigo

symptoms, allowing individuals to regain their balance and quality of life.
- Improved quality of life: By reducing vertigo symptoms, surgical treatments can improve overall quality of life and reduce the impact of vertigo on daily activities.
- Long-term relief: In some cases, surgical treatments can provide long-term relief from vertigo symptoms, eliminating the need for ongoing medication or other treatments.

What to Expect During Surgery

The specific details of your surgery will depend on the type of procedure being performed and your individual health needs. In general, surgical treatments for vertigo are performed under general anesthesia, meaning you will be asleep during the procedure. Your surgeon will provide you with specific instructions on how to prepare for surgery, including any medications you should stop taking before the procedure.

Illustrations

Here are some illustrations to help you visualize the surgical treatments for vertigo:

- Endolymphatic Sac Decompression:

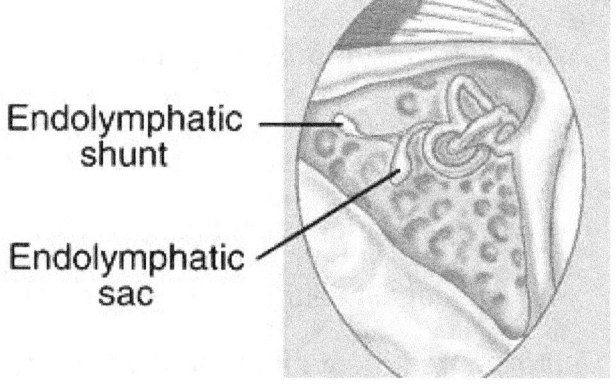

- Vestibular Nerve Section:

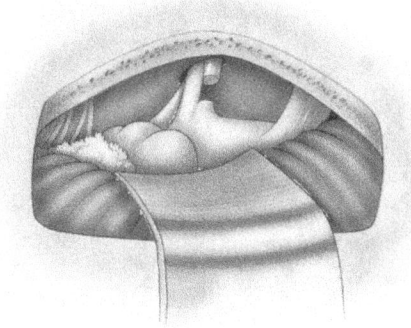

- Labyrinthectomy:

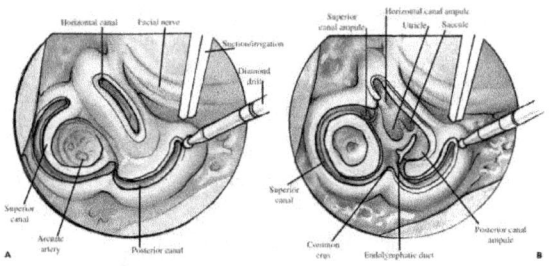

(entokey.com)

- Canal Plugging:

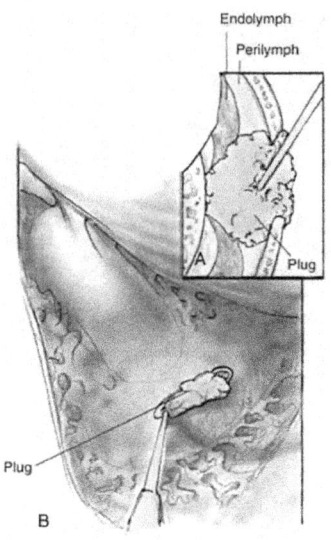

(ScienceDirect.com)

Chapter 16

Assistive Devices for Vertigo:

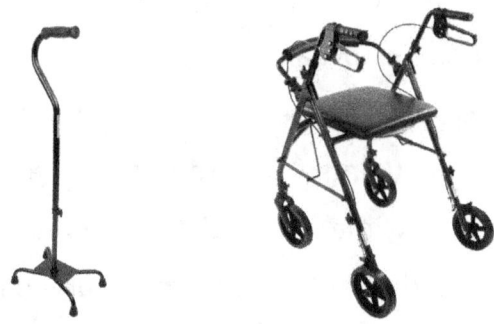

Living with vertigo can present challenges, especially when it comes to maintaining safety and independence in daily activities. Thankfully, assistive devices offer valuable support to individuals managing vertigo, enhancing stability, mobility, and overall quality of life. There are various types of assistive devices designed to address specific needs and situations, each playing a crucial role in helping vertigo patients navigate their environment with confidence and security.

One common type of assistive device for vertigo patients is the cane. Canes provide stability and support while walking, helping to reduce the risk of falls and providing a sense of security. Canes come in different styles and designs, including standard straight canes, quad canes with four small feet for added stability, and offset canes with a curved handle for improved grip and comfort. The choice of cane depends on individual preferences, balance abilities, and mobility needs. Using a cane can help vertigo patients maintain balance and stability while walking on uneven terrain or in crowded environments, enhancing safety and preventing accidents.

Another essential assistive device for vertigo patients is the walker. Walkers provide more substantial support and stability than canes, making them ideal for individuals with significant balance impairments or mobility limitations. Walkers typically feature four legs with rubber tips for traction and stability, along with hand grips for comfortable handling. Some walkers also come with wheels to facilitate smoother movement. Using a walker allows vertigo patients to navigate indoors and outdoors with greater confidence, reducing the risk of falls and providing support during activities of daily living. Walkers can be especially beneficial for individuals recovering from vestibular rehabilitation or managing chronic vestibular disorders, helping them maintain independence and mobility.

In addition to canes and walkers, vestibular patients can benefit from specialized devices designed to enhance safety and stability in specific situations. For example, balance boards and wobble cushions can be used as part of vestibular rehabilitation exercises to improve balance and proprioception. These devices challenge the vestibular system and help patients regain control over their movements. Similarly, **grab bars** and **handrails** installed in bathrooms and other high-risk areas can provide additional support and prevent slips and falls. Bed rails and bed assist handles can also help vertigo patients safely get in and out of bed, reducing the risk of injury.

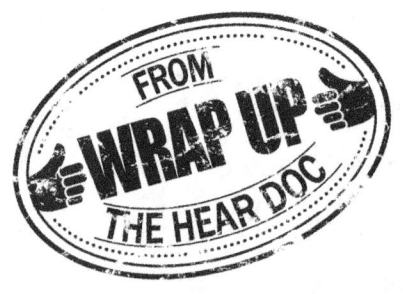

The importance of assistive devices for vertigo patients **cannot be overstated**. These devices play a vital role in promoting safety, independence, and quality of life for individuals managing vertigo and balance disorders. By providing support, stability, and confidence, assistive devices empower vertigo patients to engage in daily activities with greater ease and peace of mind. Whether it's using a cane to navigate busy streets or relying on a walker to move around the house, these devices enable vertigo patients to live life to the fullest while minimizing the risk of accidents and injuries. Ultimately, assistive devices serve as valuable tools in the management of vertigo, helping patients maintain safety and stability in their day-to-day lives.

Chapter 17

Driving Considerations with Vertigo

Driving is a fundamental aspect of independence and mobility for many individuals, allowing them to access essential services, maintain social connections, and engage in daily activities. However, for individuals living with vertigo, driving safety becomes a critical concern due to the potential for dizziness, disorientation, and impaired balance. Understanding the importance of safety while driving for patients with vertigo is essential for both the individuals themselves and the broader community.

First and foremost, **safety while driving for patients with vertigo is crucial** to prevent accidents, injuries, and even fatalities. Vertigo can cause sudden and unpredictable sensations of spinning, lightheadedness, or loss of balance, which can significantly impair driving ability and reaction times. A vertigo-related episode while behind the wheel poses a serious risk not only to the driver but also to passengers, pedestrians, and other road users. By prioritizing safety and being aware of the potential impact of vertigo on driving performance, individuals with vertigo can help mitigate these risks and protect themselves and others on the road.

Existing laws and regulations governing driving safety vary by jurisdiction but generally require drivers to meet certain physical and cognitive standards to operate a vehicle safely. In many countries, individuals with medical conditions that may affect driving ability, including vertigo and other vestibular disorders, are required to report their condition to relevant authorities, such as the Department of Motor Vehicles (DMV) or licensing agencies. Depending on the severity and frequency of vertigo symptoms, drivers may be subject to additional assessments, restrictions, or even license suspension or revocation to ensure public safety.

Liability considerations also play a significant role in driving safety for patients with vertigo. If a driver causes an accident due to vertigo-related impairment, they may be held legally and financially responsible for any resulting injuries or damages. This could lead to civil lawsuits, insurance claims, and legal penalties, highlighting the importance of managing vertigo symptoms effectively and taking appropriate precautions while driving.

By prioritizing safety and adhering to medical advice, individuals with vertigo can help mitigate the risk of accidents and minimize potential legal consequences.

There are several indications for when driving may not be recommended at all for patients with vertigo. These include:

1. Uncontrolled Symptoms: If vertigo symptoms are frequent, severe, or unpredictable, driving may pose a significant safety risk. Individuals experiencing vertigo episodes that interfere with daily activities or require frequent medication adjustments should consult their healthcare provider before driving.

2. Medication Side Effects: Certain medications used to manage vertigo symptoms, such as vestibular suppressants or sedatives, can cause drowsiness, dizziness, or

impaired cognitive function, all of which can affect driving ability. Patients should be aware of potential medication side effects and avoid driving if they feel drowsy or disoriented.

3. History of Falls or Near Misses: A history of falls, near misses, or accidents related to vertigo or balance problems is a clear indication that driving may not be safe. Individuals with a history of such incidents should undergo a comprehensive evaluation by a healthcare provider to determine their fitness to drive.

4. **Healthcare Provider Recommendation**:
Ultimately, the decision to drive should be based on the individual's overall health, symptom severity, and medical advice. Healthcare providers, including physicians, neurologists, and otolaryngologists, can assess the patient's condition, evaluate driving

risks, and provide guidance on whether driving is safe or advisable.

In conclusion, safety while driving for patients with vertigo is of paramount importance to prevent accidents, injuries, and legal consequences. Understanding the potential impact of vertigo on driving ability, adhering to relevant laws and regulations, and seeking appropriate medical guidance are essential steps to promote safe driving practices. By prioritizing safety and taking proactive measures to manage vertigo symptoms, individuals can help protect themselves and others on the road while maintaining independence and mobility.

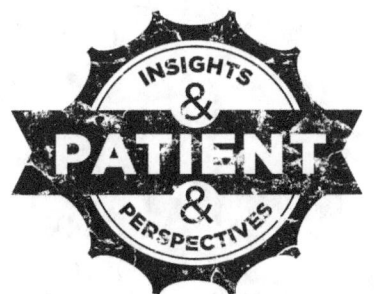

Dr. Frantz has seen several

patients with vertigo who stated that they were commercial truck drivers. It is always a difficult decision whether or not to inform the Department of Motor Vehicles of the patient's condition and place a temporary driving hold on the drivers license, but public safety and driver safety always come first. Physician reporting laws vary state by state. The driving restrictions are not necessarily permanent, but can severely affect driver income and mood.

Chapter 18

Understanding Vertigo: A Summary of Treatment Goals

Vertigo is a sensation that makes you feel like you or your surroundings are spinning or tilting, often leading to dizziness and imbalance. Although it can be quite uncomfortable, most cases are not linked to serious health issues. Here, we'll summarize the goals of treating vertigo and why it's important to see a healthcare provider.

Understanding the Cause

When you experience vertigo, the primary goal for doctors is to identify the underlying cause. They aim to determine whether the vertigo is due to a peripheral issue (usually related to the inner ear) or a central issue (related to the brain or central nervous system), as this will guide the treatment.

Timing and Triggers

Doctors will ask about:

- When the vertigo started.

- How long each episode lasts.

- Any patterns or changes over time.

- Specific actions, movements, or situations that trigger the vertigo.

This information helps categorize the type of vertigo.

Peripheral vs. Central Causes

Peripheral Causes: These typically involve problems in the inner ear or the vestibular system and are usually not serious. Conditions like benign paroxysmal positional vertigo (BPPV), Meniere's disease, and vestibular neuritis fall into this category.

Central Causes: These involve the brain or central nervous system and can be more serious, often requiring urgent attention.

Doctors use various tests, such as the HINTS examination (head-impulse, nystagmus, test of skew), to distinguish between peripheral and central causes.

Physical Examination

A thorough physical examination is essential and includes:

- Checking orthostatic blood pressure (measured when you change positions).

- Conducting a full cardiac and neurological examination.

- Assessing for nystagmus (involuntary eye movements).

- Performing the Dix-Hallpike maneuver, especially if BPPV is suspected.

Laboratory Testing and Imaging

Routine blood tests and imaging (like MRI or CT scans) are generally not needed for most vertigo cases. However, imaging may be recommended if a central cause is suspected.

Treatment Goals

The treatment plan for vertigo focuses on several key goals:

Addressing the Underlying Cause

Treatment is tailored to the specific cause of vertigo.

BPPV: The Epley maneuver, a procedure to reposition canaliths in the inner ear, can be very effective.

Meniere's Disease: A low-salt diet and diuretics can help manage fluid balance in the inner ear.

Vestibular Neuritis: Medications and vestibular rehabilitation therapy can aid recovery.

Relieving Symptoms

Medications can help manage symptoms such as nausea, dizziness, and anxiety. Common medications include antiemetics (to reduce nausea), antihistamines, and sometimes benzodiazepines.

Vestibular rehabilitation therapy (VRT) is also beneficial. This involves exercises designed to improve balance, eye movements, and overall stability during daily activities.

Supporting Recovery

Providing patients with accurate information about their condition and treatment options is crucial. Educating patients on lifestyle modifications, such as avoiding known triggers and staying hydrated, can help manage symptoms and prevent future episodes.

Importance of Seeing a Healthcare Provider

Seeing a healthcare provider is essential for several reasons:

Accurate Diagnosis: Proper evaluation can identify whether vertigo is due to a benign condition or something more serious that requires immediate attention.

Tailored Treatment: A healthcare provider can develop a treatment plan specific to the underlying cause of your vertigo, ensuring effective management.

Monitoring Progress: Regular check-ups help monitor your condition and make necessary adjustments to your treatment plan.

Education and Support: Healthcare providers can offer valuable information and support to help you cope with vertigo and improve your quality of life.

In summary, while vertigo can be a distressing symptom, understanding its causes and getting appropriate treatment can significantly improve your well-being. Always consult a healthcare provider to ensure you receive the right care.

Chapter 19

The Future of Vertigo Treatments, Diagnosis and Prevention of Falls and Injury.

Vertigo, a sensation of spinning or dizziness, significantly impacts the quality of life for many individuals. It can result from various causes, including inner ear problems, vestibular disorders, and neurological conditions. As our understanding of vertigo deepens, advancements in technology, medicine, and robotics promise to revolutionize the way vertigo is diagnosed, treated, and prevented. This chapter explores the future landscape of vertigo care, highlighting innovations in robotic assistants, medical devices, medications, and preventive strategies.

Advancements in Vertigo Testing

The future of vertigo testing is set to benefit immensely from technological advancements.

Traditional methods such as the Dix-Hallpike test and electronystagmography (ENG) are effective but have limitations. Emerging technologies offer more precise, non-invasive, and patient-friendly diagnostic tools.

Robotic Assistants in Diagnostic Procedures

Robotic systems are being developed to assist clinicians in performing precise diagnostic maneuvers. These robots can replicate movements accurately, reducing variability and human error in tests like the Dix-Hallpike maneuver. Moreover, robotic systems can be equipped with sensors to provide real-time feedback on a patient's condition, enhancing the accuracy of vertigo diagnosis.

Advanced Imaging Techniques

Future imaging techniques, such as high-resolution MRI and vestibular functional

MRI, will allow clinicians to visualize inner ear structures and brain activity in unprecedented detail. These methods can identify subtle abnormalities that might be missed with current imaging technologies. Additionally, portable imaging devices are in development, enabling point-of-care diagnostics, especially beneficial in remote or underserved areas.

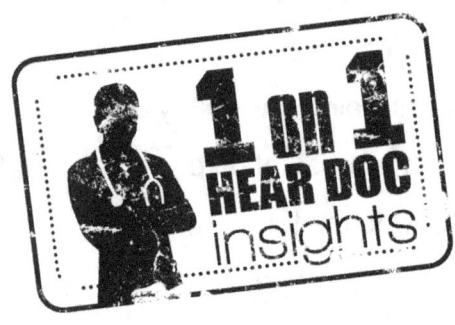

Wearable Diagnostic Devices

Wearable technology, such as smart glasses and head-mounted sensors, will play a crucial role in vertigo diagnostics. These devices can monitor eye movements, head position, and balance in real-time, providing continuous data that can help in early detection and monitoring of vertigo symptoms.

Integration with artificial intelligence (AI) algorithms will enable the analysis of large datasets to identify patterns and **predict** vertigo episodes.

Innovations in Vertigo Treatment

The treatment of vertigo is poised to undergo significant transformations with the integration of AI inclusive robotics, advanced medical devices, and novel medications.

Robotic Vestibular Rehabilitation

Vestibular rehabilitation therapy (VRT) is a cornerstone in managing vertigo, particularly for conditions like benign paroxysmal positional vertigo (BPPV) and vestibular neuritis. Robotic systems using AI can enhance VRT by providing precise, repetitive, and customizable exercises that target specific vestibular deficits. These robots can adapt to a patient's progress, ensuring optimal rehabilitation outcomes.

Personalized Medication Regimens

Advances in pharmacogenomics will allow for personalized medication regimens tailored to an individual's genetic profile. This approach will minimize side effects and maximize efficacy, particularly important for medications used to treat vertigo, such as vestibular suppressants and antiemetics. Furthermore, new classes of drugs targeting specific pathways involved in vertigo are being developed, promising more effective and faster relief.

Implantable Devices

Implantable vestibular devices, such as the vestibular implant, are on the horizon. 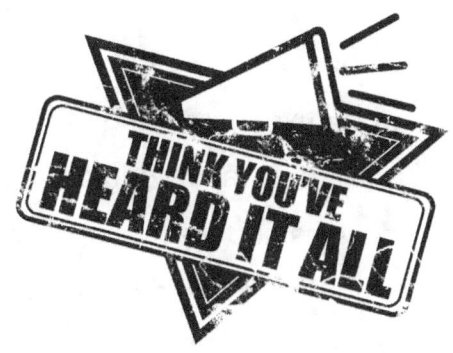 These devices function similarly to cochlear implants but target the vestibular system. They can restore balance function in patients with severe bilateral vestibular loss, offering a transformative solution for those with debilitating vertigo.

Preventive Strategies for Vertigo

Preventing vertigo involves addressing underlying causes, enhancing early detection, and implementing lifestyle modifications.

Proactive Monitoring and Early Intervention

AI-powered predictive analytics will enable proactive monitoring of individuals at risk for vertigo. By analyzing data from wearable devices and electronic health records, AI algorithms can identify early warning signs and trigger preventive interventions. This approach can prevent the progression of vertigo or reduce the severity of episodes.

Lifestyle Modifications and Education

Public health initiatives will focus on educating individuals about lifestyle factors that can contribute to vertigo, such as diet, hydration, and stress management. Virtual reality (VR) platforms can provide immersive educational experiences, helping individuals understand their condition and adopt healthier habits.

Genetic Screening and Counseling

Genetic screening for hereditary vestibular disorders will become more accessible and affordable. Early identification of genetic predispositions can inform preventive strategies and enable individuals to take proactive steps to manage their risk.

The future of vertigo care is bright, with numerous innovations on the horizon. Robotic assistants, advanced diagnostic devices, personalized medications, and preventive strategies will transform the way vertigo is managed. These advancements promise to enhance the accuracy of diagnosis, the efficacy of treatment, and the effectiveness of preventive measures, ultimately improving the quality of life for individuals affected by vertigo. As technology continues to evolve, the integration of these innovations into clinical practice will usher in a new era of vertigo care.

Chapter 20

Final Thoughts

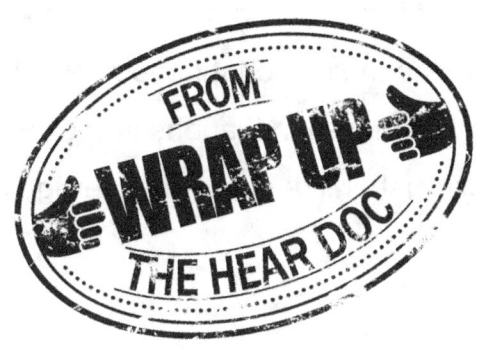

Remember, most cases of vertigo are not serious, but proper evaluation and targeted treatment can significantly improve your quality of life. If you experience persistent or severe vertigo, consult a healthcare professional for personalized guidance. The future of vertigo care is bright, with numerous innovations on the horizon. Robotic assistants, advanced diagnostic devices, personalized medications, and preventive strategies will transform the way vertigo is managed. These advancements promise to enhance the accuracy of diagnosis, the efficacy of treatment, and the effectiveness of preventive measures, ultimately improving the quality of life for individuals affected by vertigo. As technology continues to evolve, the integration of these innovations into clinical practice will usher in a new era of vertigo care.

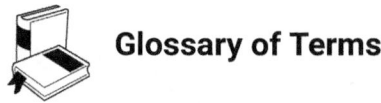 **Glossary of Terms**

Acoustic Nerve: transmits nerve impulses from the cochlea to the brain.

Acoustic Neuroma: a tumor of the acoustic nerve which creates hearing loss, vertigo and tinnitus and is usually not cancerous.

BTE: a type of hearing aid worn Behind-The-Ear.

Cerumen: also known as earwax.

Cholesteatoma: an abnormal growth of skin cells in the middle ear and mastoid.

Cochlea: the tiny inner ear, snail shell shaped structure which transforms mechanical sound energy into electrical nerve impulses.

Conductive Hearing Loss: a type of hearing loss which prevents sound wave energy from reaching the cochlea.

Custom hearing aid: a type of hearing aid which is worn in the ear which often requires an ear mold impression to be made for a proper fit.

Dizziness: a term used to describe a range of sensations, such as feeling faint, woozy, lightheaded, weak or unsteady.

Incus: the ossicle which connects the malleus bone to the stapes bone.

Labyrinth: an inner ear system which controls balance also called the semicircular canals.

Malleus: the ossicle which connects the tympanic membrane to the incus bone.

Microphone: the part of a hearing aid which picks up sound. One or two may be present on each hearing aid.

Mixed Hearing Loss: a type of hearing loss which has both conductive and sensorineural components.

Ossicles: the three tiny bones in the middle ear that conduct sound energy.

Ossiculoplasty: a procedure to replace or repair missing or damaged ossicles.

RITE (or RIC): a type of hearing aid worn on or behind the ear which has the speaker in the ear canal also called Receiver-In-The-Ear.

Saccule: inner ear organ senses gravitational acceleration.

Semicircular canals: Inner ear organs which sense rotational acceleration.

Sensorineural Hearing Loss: a type of hearing loss in which sounds are not processed in the cochlea or not transmitted to the brain correctly through the acoustic nerve.

Stapes: the smallest of the ossicles which connects the incus to the cochlea.

Tinnitus: a sound heard in the ear(s) which is not present in a person's environment.

Tympanic Membrane: also known as the eardrum. It conducts sounds from the environment to the ossicles

Utricle: an inner ear organ which senses gravitational acceleration.

Vertigo: a sensation of motion often associated with loss of balance, usually caused by disease affecting the inner ear or the vestibular nerve

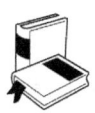 **References:**

- https://my.clevelandclinic.org/health/diseases/21769-vertigo
- Merriam-Webster's Dictionary
- https://www.ncbi.nlm.nih.gov/pmc/articles/PMC6873344/
- https://preventous.com/the-importance-of-being-balanced/
- https://www.betterhealth.vic.gov.au/health/conditionsandtreatments/dizziness-and-vertigo
- https://journals.sagepub.com/doi/10.1177/0269215507082741
- https://vestibular.org/article/what-is-vestibular/the-human-balance-system/the-human-balance-system-how-do-we-maintain-our-balance/
- https://www.informedhealth.org/
- https://www.ncbi.nlm.nih.gov/pmc/articles/PMC9428313/
- Robbins S, Gouw GJ, McClaran J. Shoe sole thickness and hardness influence

balance in older men. J Am Geriatr Soc. 1992;40(11):1089-94.

- [ ] Perry SD, Radtke A, Goodwin CR. Influence of footwear midsole material hardness on dynamic balance control during unexpected gait termination. Gait Posture. 2007; 25(1):94-98.

- [ ] https://vestibular.org/article/coping-support/living-with-a-vestibular-disorder/footwear/

- [ ] https://www.semanticscholar.org/paper/The-influence-of-high-heeled-shoes-on-balance-and-Weon-Cha/d136439c90d09abd84752dab1659ad27c111c16c

- [ ] Kim J-S, Zee DS. Benign Paroxysmal Positional Vertigo. *N Engl J Med*. 2014; 370(12): p.1138-1147

- [ ] Muncie HL, Sirmans SM, James E. Dizziness: Approach to Evaluation and Management.. *Am Fam Physician*. 2017; 95(3): p.154-162. pmid: 28145669.

- [ ] Kim J-S. When the Room Is Spinning: Experience of Vestibular Neuritis by a Neurotologist. *Front Neurol*. 2020; 11. doi: 10.3389/fneur.2020.00157

- [ ] Halmagyi, G. M., & Curthoys, I. S. (2016). Vestibular neuritis: clinical features and diagnosis. Journal of Neurology, Neurosurgery & Psychiatry, 87(3), 294-298.

- [ ] Basura GJ, Adams ME, Monfared A, et al. Clinical Practice Guideline: Ménière's Disease. *Otolaryngol Head Neck Surg*. 2020; 162(2_suppl): p.S1-S55. doi: 10.1177/0194599820909438

- [ ] Lopez-Escamez, J. A., et al. (2015). Diagnostic criteria for Menière's disease. Journal of Vestibular Research: Equilibrium & Orientation, 25(1), 1-7.

- [ ] Dieterich, M., & Obermann, M. (2019). Vestibular migraine: the most frequent entity of episodic vertigo. Journal of Neurology, 266(1), 82-89.

- [ ] Hilton DB, Lui F, Shermetaro C. Migraine-Associated Vertigo. [Updated 2024 Feb 12]. In: StatPearls [Internet]. Treasure Island (FL): StatPearls Publishing; 2024 Jan-. Available from: https://www.ncbi.nlm.nih.gov/books/NBK507859/

- [ ] Stangerup, S. E., Cayé-Thomasen, P., & Tos, M. (2010). True incidence of vestibular schwannoma? Neurosurgery, 67(5), 1335-1340.

- [ ] Kerber, K. A., & Brown, D. L. (2014). Stroke risk stratification in acute dizziness presentations: a prospective imaging-based study. Neurology, 83(6), 495-501.

- [ ] Halmagyi, G. M., & Aw, S. T. (2006). Advances in pharmacological management of vestibular disorders. Journal of Neurology, 253(3), 305-313.

- [ ] Scherer, M. R., et al. (2011). Traumatic brain injury and vestibular pathology as a comorbidity after blast exposure. Physical Therapy, 91(8), 1153-1163.

- [ ] https://www.mayoclinic.org/diseases-conditions/dizziness/symptoms-causes/syc-20371787

- [ ] Strupp, M., et al. (2021). Vestibular disorders of central origin. Handbook of Clinical Neurology, 175, 123-134.

- [ ] Newman-Toker, D. E., & Kerber, K. A. (2008). HINTS to diagnose stroke in the acute vestibular syndrome: three-step bedside oculomotor examination more sensitive than early MRI diffusion-weighted imaging. Stroke, 39(11), 3024-3030.

☐ Lee, H., & Sohn, S. I. (2013). Timing of atrial fibrillation and flutter relative to symptoms and ECG. Journal of Neurology, Neurosurgery & Psychiatry, 84(7), 706-709.

☐ Strupp M, et al. "Peripheral vestibular disorders." Handbook of Clinical Neurology, 2016; 137:317-334.

☐ Singh R, et al. "Ophthalmologic causes of dizziness and vertigo." Journal of Neuro-Ophthalmology, 2020; 40(1):88-97.

☐ Lee H. "Neuro-otological aspects of migraine." Journal of Clinical Neurology, 2010; 6(2):57-63.

☐ Agrawal Y, et al. "Dizziness: A Diagnostic Approach." American Journal of Medicine, 2010; 123(9):724-728.

☐ Hillier, S. L., & McDonnell, M. (2011). Vestibular rehabilitation for unilateral peripheral vestibular dysfunction. Cochrane Database of Systematic Reviews, 2, CD005397.

☐ Ruckenstein, M. J., Staab, J. P., & Newman-Toker, D. E. (2009). Dopamine agonists and anticholinergics in the treatment of vestibular disorders. Current Treatment Options in Neurology, 11(1), 41–45.

☐ Hilton, M. P., Pinder, D. K., & The, D. S. (2014). The Epley (canalith repositioning) manoeuvre for benign paroxysmal positional vertigo. Cochrane Database of Systematic Reviews, 12, CD003162.

☐ Hall, C. D., et al. (2016). Exercise for the treatment of neurological disorders: a systematic review. Clinical Rehabilitation, 30(8), 795–807.

☐ Dai M, et al. "Dietary factors associated with migraine and tension-type headache in China: A case-control study." Nutr Neurosci. 2017; 20(6):1-8.

☐ Ryan C, et al. "Dietary factors and the incidence of vertigo and dizziness in

American adults." Nutrients. 2019; 11(1):190

☐ Cha YH, et al. "Effects of caffeine on vestibular function among patients with vestibular migraine." Neurology. 2016; 86(18):1713-9.

☐ Cha YH, et al. "Effects of caffeine on vestibular function among patients with vestibular migraine." Neurology. 2016; 86(18):1713-9.

☐ Strupp M, et al. "Vestibular migraine: Diagnostic criteria." J Vestib Res. 2012; 22(4):167-72.

☐ Hillier S, McDonnell M. "Vestibular rehabilitation for unilateral peripheral vestibular dysfunction." Cochrane Database Syst Rev. 2011; (2):CD005397.

☐ Bhattacharyya N, et al. "Clinical practice guideline: benign paroxysmal positional vertigo." Otolaryngol Head Neck Surg. 2017; 156(3_suppl):S1-S47.

☐ McDonnell MN, Hillier SL. "Vestibular rehabilitation for unilateral peripheral vestibular dysfunction." Cochrane Database Syst Rev. 2015; (1):CD005397.

- [ ] Pullens B, van Benthem PP. "Surgery for Ménière's disease." Cochrane Database Syst Rev. 2013; (2):CD005395.
- [ ] Committee on Hearing and Equilibrium guidelines for the diagnosis and evaluation of therapy in Menière's disease. American Academy of Otolaryngology-Head and Neck Foundation, Inc. Otolaryngol Head Neck Surg. 1995; 113(3):181-5.
- [ ] Ishiyama G, Ishiyama A. "Canal occlusion surgery for benign paroxysmal positional vertigo: a review." Acta Otolaryngol. 2014; 134(6):558-65.
- [ ] Lee JD, Kim CH, Hong SM, Park CH. "Long-term outcome of endolymphatic sac surgery for intractable Meniere's disease." Acta Otolaryngol. 2011; 131(1):26-30.

Check out other publications by The Hear Doc ™

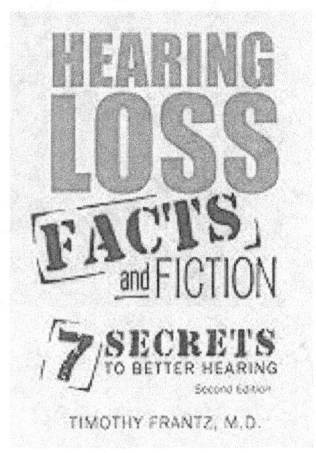

Hearing Loss: Facts and Fiction: 7 Secrets to Better Hearing

by Timothy Frantz M.D. | Feb 18, 2015

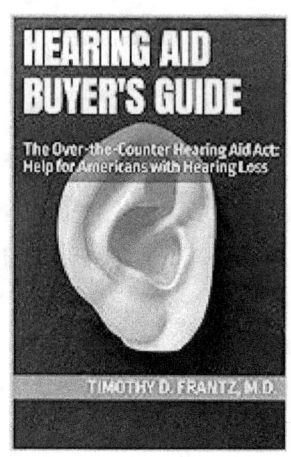

Hearing Aid Buyer's Guide: The Over-the-Counter Hearing Aid Act: Help for Americans with Hearing Loss

by Timothy Frantz M.D. | Nov 22, 2022

About the Authors:

Timothy Frantz, MD (The Hear Doc ™) is a board-certified Otolaryngologist/ Head and Neck Surgeon (ENT) with over 30 years of experience in the treatment of ear disease and general Otolaryngology. Dr. Frantz attended RFU / The Chicago Medical School, where he serves as a medical student mentor in Otolaryngology. In addition to private practice in Pennsylvania, he also serves as a U.S. Navy Reserves Medical Officer. He has authored several publications in major medical journals, and has lectured nationally on various ENT topics.

Matthew Kim, MD is a recent graduate of RFU / The Chicago Medical School and is currently working as an Otolaryngology resident surgeon at Southern Illinois University in Springfield, Illinois. In addition to this book, he has authored several scientific publications and has a profound interest in Otolaryngology/Head and Neck Surgery.

If you have further questions, or wish to be on our email list for future health related publications, please reach out to the authors at:

Vertigorxbook@gmail.com

www.ingramcontent.com/pod-product-compliance
Lightning Source LLC
Chambersburg PA
CBHW050057230526
45470CB00004B/1566